"Freud's *Moses and Monotheism* was begun in the wake of the rise of Nazi anti-semitism in Europe and completed towards the end of his life. The Editor, Lawrence J. Brown, states it is a 'fascinating, controversial, quirky, and ultimately thought-provoking work' that is relevant to many of the social and cultural issues that we struggle with today. This volume, written by an outstanding international cast of psychoanalysts and scholars, not only offers contemporary readers a window into Freud's personal biography and final thoughts, but explicates and extends Freud's understanding of a wide range of topics from large group dynamics and the nature of leadership and religion to Biblical/ethnographic studies and, of course, addresses many topics of psychoanalytic interest, including phylogenesis, metapsychology, the intergenerational transmission of trauma, the nature of memory, historical truth and psychical reality, and the origins of neurosis in the individual and society. The depth and intelligence of this volume promises to restore Freud's final book contribution to its rightful place as a testament to the continued relevance of his insights and intuitions."

Howard B. Levine, MD, Editor-in-Chief,
Routledge W.R. Bion Studies Series

"Freud's works are an inexhaustible source of inspiration and knowledge. In *On Freud's 'Moses and Monotheism,'* Lawrence J. Brown offers a selection of fascinating writings on what can be considered Freud's most personal book, the one that reveals his passions and torments. The fact that *Moses and Monotheism* is such a controversial, flawed, and in many ways obscure book becomes a richer asset due to the multitude of contemporary interpretations that lurk in the folds of this last 'non-analytic' child of Freud. The authors, psychoanalysts from different parts of the world, each offer their own Moses and their own Freud. The reader thus has the opportunity to meet living and contemporary characters, who give this classic a new surprising vitality. I highly recommend reading *On Freud's 'Moses and Monotheism'* to all psychoanalysts, scholars of humanities, and anyone who is interested in psychoanalytic thought."

Giuseppe Civitarese, author, *Sublime Subjects: Aesthetic Experience and Intersubjectivity in Psychoanalysis*

"Of all the books and articles that constitute Freud's legacy, his late work *Moses and Monotheism* is perhaps one of the most puzzling and, as such, difficult to master... or to ignore. Unsurprisingly, it has been controversial from the start, showing, for one thing, that old age did not diminish Freud's courage. His last great work, indeed, has not finished asking difficult questions – to humankind, to psychoanalysis, and to each of us, if we accept to enter its complex structure and to ponder the exigency it exerts on our minds. The notion of 'historical truth,' for one, raises issues that lay at the center of our idea of civilization. The present book, edited by Lawrence J. Brown, offers us the helping hand of a series of excellent contributions from international authors who enlighten and question us in the Freudian spirit. It is a welcome companion in this adventure in thinking."

Dominique Scarfone, author, *The Unpast: The Actual Unconscious*

On Freud's "Moses and Monotheism"

On Freud's "Moses and Monotheism" discusses key themes in Sigmund Freud's final book, *Moses and Monotheism,* written between 1934 and 1939. The contributors reflect on the historical context of the time during which the book was written, including Freud's mindset and his struggle to leave Austria to escape the Nazi regime, and investigate its contemporary implications and relevance.

Drawing parallels with contemporary society, the chapters cover topics like historical truth, the effects of Nazism on Freud's writing, Freud's "relationship" with Moses, the transmission of trauma across generations, the origins and psychodynamics of anti-Semitism, Freud and Moses as leaders, and the notion of Tradition. This book also reflects on the stories of Moses and of Freud – the search of a people for a "Promised Land," the deep scars of slavery, and the struggle of a man to establish an ideology and ensure its continuity.

On Freud's "Moses and Monotheism" will be of great interest to all psychoanalysts and psychoanalytic psychotherapists. It will also be of interest to scholars investigating the nature of truth, and social scientists interested in the broader applications of Freud's discussions of the nature of civilization.

Lawrence J. Brown is trained in adult and child psychoanalysis and is a faculty member and supervising child analyst at the Boston Psychoanalytic Institute, USA. He is also a supervising and personal analyst at the Massachusetts Institute for Psychoanalysis. Brown has lectured internationally and published papers on a variety of topics, including the Oedipal situation, Bion, intersubjectivity, field theory, and autistic phenomena.

The International Psychoanalytical Association
Contemporary Freud Turning Points and Critical Issues Series

Series Editor: Gabriela Legorreta

On Freud's "Observations on Transference-Love"
Edited by Ethel Spector Person, Aiban Hagelin, Peter Fonagy

On Freud's "Creative Writers and Day-Dreaming"
Edited by Ethel Spector Person, Peter Fonagy, Sérvulo Augusto Figueira

On Freud's "A Child Is Being Beaten"
Edited by Ethel Spector Person

On Freud's "Analysis Terminable and Interminable"
Edited by Joseph Sandler

On Freud's "The Unconscious"
Edited by Salman Akhtar and Mary Kay O'Neil

On Freud's "Screen Memories"
Edited by Gail S. Reed and Howard B. Levine

On Freud's "Formulations on the Two Principles of Mental Functioning"
Edited by Gabriela Legorreta and Lawrence J. Brown

On Freud's "The Question of Lay Analysis"
Edited by Paulo Cesar Sandler and Gley Pacheco Costa

On Freud's "The Uncanny"
Edited by Catalina Bronstein and Christian Seulin

On Freud's "Moses and Monotheism"
Edited by Lawrence J. Brown

On Freud's "Moses and Monotheism"

Edited by Lawrence J. Brown

Routledge
Taylor & Francis Group
LONDON AND NEW YORK

Cover image: Freud by Julia Kotulova, charcoal & digital, 2019

First published 2023
by Routledge
4 Park Square, Milton Park, Abingdon, Oxon OX14 4RN

and by Routledge
605 Third Avenue, New York, NY 10158

Routledge is an imprint of the Taylor & Francis Group, an informa business

British Library Cataloguing-in-Publication Data
A catalogue record for this book is available from the British Library

ISBN: 9781032223124 (hbk)
ISBN: 9781032223131 (pbk)
ISBN: 9781003272045 (ebk)

DOI: 10.4324/9781003272045

Typeset in Palatino
by Newgen Publishing UK

I dedicate this book to my wife, Fran Brown, for her support and perseverance.

Contents

Contributors

David Benhaim trained as psychoanalyst at the Canadian Psychoanalytic Society and has a philosophical background. He is a psychoanalyst *habilité*. He has published numerous articles in the *Canadian Journal of Psychoanalysis*, in the French journals *Topique, Cliniques méditerranéennes, Enfance & psy, Le Divan familial*, in the Quebec journal *Filigrane* and in the Argentine journal *Psicoanálisis e intersubjetividad* of which he is the technical advisor. From 2011 to 2016 he was co-editor of the *Psychoanalytic Journal of Couple and Family* of the *International Psychoanalytic Association of Couple and Family* (IPACF). He has participated in several collectives such as *Actualités de l'événement* (Editor Liber), *La survivance en heritage* (Editor Presses de l'Université Laval). He is also member of the reading committee of the journal *Le Divan familial* of Paris.

Rachel B. Blass is a Training and Supervising Analyst at the Israel Psychoanalytic Society, a member of the British Psychoanalytical Society, on the Board of the *International Journal of Psychoanalysis* where she is the editor of the Controversies section. She was formerly a professor of psychoanalysis at universities both in Israel and England. She has published a book and numerous papers that elucidate the foundations of analytic thinking and practice, with a special focus on Kleinian psychoanalysis and its Freudian roots. Her writings have been translated into 15 languages. While she lives and practices in Jerusalem, via the internet she also teaches and supervises in the US, Australia, and several countries in Europe and Asia.

Sara Boffito is an IPA Psychoanalyst and Children and Adolescents Psychoanalyst, and member of the Italian Psychoanalytic Society. She is Associate Editor of the *International Journal of Psychoanalysis*, member of the editorial board of *Rivista di Psicoanalisi* (Journal of the Italian Psychoanalytic Society) and of the *COWAP IPA Book Series* (Routledge) editorial board. Besides publishing and presenting several works in international journals, congresses, and collective books, she also translates foundational English language authors of psychoanalysis into Italian.

Lawrence Brown, PhD is Editor of this book. He is a graduate and faculty member of the Boston Psychoanalytic Institute in child and adult psychoanalysis and is a supervising child analyst. He is also a faculty member and personal analyst at the Massachusetts Institute for Psychoanalysis. He has published extensively and lectured internationally on such topics as trauma, the Oedipal situation, intersubjectivity, the work of Bion, Klein, and autistic phenomena. He has published several books: Brown, L. J. (2011) *Intersubjective Processes and the Unconscious: An Integration of Freudian, Kleinian and Bionian Perspectives* Routledge; Levine, H. & Brown, L. J. (2013) *Growth and Turbulence in the Container/Contained: Bion's Continuing Legacy.* Routledge; Legoretta, G. & Brown, L. J. (2016) *On Freud's "Formulations on the Two Principles of Mental Functioning"* London: Karnac; and Brown, L. J. (2019) *Transformational Processes in Clinical Psychoanalysis: Dreaming, Emotions and the Present Moment.* Routledge.

Sara Collins is a Training and Supervising Psychoanalyst at the British Psychoanalytic Association, and a past Director of Training at the BPA. She is the Book Reviews Editor of the *International Journal of Psychoanalysis* and a board member of *The Psychoanalytic Quarterly.* A contributor to a number of books, she has given papers and published on memory and its construction in psychoanalysis and literature, and on theory of psychoanalytic practice, including on analysts' enactments as memories. She holds roles on committees concerned with psychoanalytic education, as well as the Programme Committee of the European Psychoanalytic Federation.

Shmuel Erlich is a Training and Supervising Analyst and past President of the Israel Psychoanalytic Society. He was Sigmund Freud Professor of Psychoanalysis (Emeritus) and Director of the Sigmund Freud Center at The Hebrew University of Jerusalem. He chaired the IPA Education Committee, served four terms as European Representative on the IPA Board, and is currently Chair of the IPA Institutional Issues Committee. He received the Sigourney Award for outstanding contributions to psychoanalysis in 2005. His publications span adolescent development and psychopathology, experiential dimensions of object relations, group and organizational processes, and two books: *The Couch in the Marketplace: Psychoanalysis and Social Reality*, and *Fed with Tears, Poisoned with Milk: Germans and Israelis, The Past in the Present*. He is in private practice in Tel Aviv.

Peter T. Hoffer, PhD, is Emeritus Professor of German at the University of the Sciences in an Educator Associate of the American Psychoanalytic

Association. He is co-translator (with Axel Hoffer) of Sigmund Freud's *A Phylogenetic Fantasy: Overview of the Transference Neuroses* and translator of the three-volume *Correspondence of Sigmund Freud and Sandor Ferenczi* and Richard Sterba's *Handwörterbuch der Psychoanalyse* (Dictionary of Psychoanalysis). He is also the author of several published papers on the history of psychoanalysis.

Laurence Kahn worked as an historian and anthropologist of Ancient Greece before becoming a psychoanalyst. Now a Training and Supervising Analyst at the French Psychoanalytic Association (APF), she was co-editor of the *Nouvelle Revue de Psychanalyse* from 1990 to 1994. Dividing her time between practice, training, and writing, she held the function of President of the APF from 2008 to 2010, and was the Editor in Chief of *L'Annuel de l'APF* from 2010 to 2015. She has also written several books in French and a forthcoming book translated book, *What Nazism Did to Psychoanalysis*, Routledge). And numerous articles in journals and collections of essays in France and abroad, such as "If only one knew *what* exists!" (*Unrepresented States and the Construction of Meaning*, Levine, Reed & Scarfone ed., Karnac, 2013).

Eran J. Rolnik, MD, PhD, is a psychiatrist, historian, and training and supervising analyst and on the faculty of the Israel Psychoanalytic Society and Institute. In addition to numerous journal papers and chapters in edited volumes he translated and edited several volumes with Freud's essays and published three monographs: *Freud in Zion: Psychoanalysis and the Making of Modern Jewish Identity* (Karnac 2012]; *Sigmund Freud Letters* (Modan 2019); *A Talking Cure: 13 talks on Psychoanalysis* (Carmel 2022).

Merav Roth, PhD, is a clinical psychologist and a training and supervising psychoanalyst at the Israeli psychoanalytic society; She is the head of the psychoanalytic psychotherapy program, Sackler school of Medicine, Tel-Aviv University; and a researcher of the interdisciplinary link between psychoanalysis and culture (mainly literature). She is the former chair of the interdisciplinary Doctoral program in psychoanalysis and the former founder and chair of the post graduate Klein studies, both at the psychoanalytic psychotherapy program, Sackler school of Medicine, Tel-Aviv University. Together with Joshua Durban, Roth edited and wrote the Preface and introductions to the book *Melanie Klein – Essential Papers II* (Tel Aviv: Book-Worm, 2013) and also edited Klein's *Psychoanalysis of Children* (Tel Aviv: Book-Worm, in press) and Brenman Pick's *Authenticity in the Psychoanalytic Encounter* (Jerusalem: Carmel, 2021). Her book *Reading the Reader – a Psychoanalytic Perspective on Literature* was published by Routledge (London and New York: Routledge, 2020) and is nowadays translated into Spanish.

Series Editor's Foreword

This series, "Contemporary Freud, Turning Points and Critical Issues," was founded in 1991 by Robert Wallerstein and subsequently edited by Joseph Sandler, Ethel Spector Person, Peter Fonagy, Leticia Glocer Fiorini and recently by Gennaro Saragnano. The books published in this Series have greatly interested psychoanalysts from different regions and have succeeded at creating a new modality of exchange. It is therefore my great honor, as Chair of the Publications Committee of the International Psychoanalytic Association, to continue the tradition of this most successful series.

The objective of this series is to approach Freud's work both from a historical and a contemporary point of view. On the one hand, this means highlighting the fundamental contributions of his work that constitute the axes of psychoanalytic theory and practice. On the other, it implies learning about and presenting the understanding of Freud's oeuvre of present psychoanalysts, both where they coincide and where they differ.

In this Series one appreciates that Freud's papers present ideas that still merit discussion and also elaboration. The expansion of his work by present day analysts is a testimony to the richness of his legacy with its originality, creativity and at times, provocative thinking. His work has become a breeding ground from which new ideas and developments have arisen.

Freud's theory has been extended, and this has led to a theoretical, technical, and clinical pluralism that must be understood by students of psychoanalysis. It is necessary to avoid a comfortable, uncritical coexistence of concepts and to contemplate systems of increasing complexity.

This Series gathers psychoanalysts from different geographical regions with different theoretical stances, to be able to show their polyphony. This requires an effort on the part of the reader to distinguish, discriminate and establish relations or contradictions to eventually work through the significance of Freud's papers.

In this volume Lawrence Brown brings together contributors from different regions of the IPA, whose papers are a testimony to the importance and value of Freud's last book: *Moses and Monotheism*. The chapters deal with a variety of themes that enlighten Freud's, at times, debatable ideas expressed in this book.

One of the themes which is explored by three contributors is the connection between Freud's paper and the rise of Nazism that forced him to emigrate to London. In her chapter, Laurence Kahn emphasizes the way in which hatred was rampant and the law, either Moses' Tables of the Law or secular law, was perverted in an attempt to purify German society following Nazi principles of German superiority. In his concluding remarks Lawrence Brown also offers his perspective on how Nazism influenced Freud in some of the ideas developed in his last book. Sara Bofitto also examines this subject by discussing Freud's hesitations in publishing *Moses and Monotheism* due to the unsafe atmosphere and danger during Nazi occupation.

Another important subject examined in this volume is that of Phylogenetic Fantasy and the reappearance of repressed memories from our ancient histories. This topic is addressed by Peter Hoffer as well as David Benahim who examines this question through his discussion of the origin and nature of tradition, claiming that the reason for the disappearance of some traditions and their reappearance after a long period of inertia can be explained through the return of the repressed. The most important and intriguing notion of historical truth is also examined.

Another subject studied by a few contributors such as Merav Roth, Lawrence Brown, and Erlich Shmuel is Freud's deep identification with Moses, beginning with his reverence for the prophet during childhood. For some of these authors, this identification implies that, just as Moses has received the Torah from God and is responsible for cultivating and guarding its teachings, so Freud has created psychoanalysis as a comparable discipline that is fostered and taught around the world. Erlich Shmuel addresses this subject by introducing the reader to Freud's notion of The Great Man, that is, men who have an extraordinary capacity to gather individuals and families and determine their destiny. In this regard, Erlich Shmuel argues, Freud and Moses are both Great Men.

The Publications Committee is pleased to publish this book, *On Freud's "Moses and Monotheism,"* which constitutes the 20th volume of the IPA "Contemporary Freud Turning Points and Critical Issues" series. Lawrence Brown has brilliantly and skilfully edited this new volume. He selected nine distinguished colleagues from different regions to discuss and re-consider Freud's ideas in the light of contemporary psychoanalytic thinking. The result is this important book, which will surely encounter the favour of every student of psychoanalysis as well as of others interested in Freud's work and its evolution as well as the complexity of mental life. I want to thank wholeheartedly the editor and contributors of this new volume, which continues the tradition of the IPA book series.

Gabriela Legorreta
Series Editor
Chair, IPA Publications Committee

Editor's Introduction to *On Freud's "Moses and Monotheism"*

Lawrence J. Brown

This book is being published by the International Psychoanalytic Association Publications Committee through its Contemporary Freud Series in which each volume consists of various authors' essays in response to one of Freud's papers, with an emphasis on the contemporary relevance to the papers. Each of the volumes begins with a reprint of Freud's original paper and followed by the chapters written by the contributors. However, *Moses and Monotheism* is quite long (138 pages) and so including it in its entirety is unrealistic given the page limitations for each book in the series. One option was to reduce the length of the chapters and include the entire *Moses and Monotheism*, but this choice would unnecessarily constrain the authors; consequently, it was decided that the Editor (LJB) would write a brief introduction to each chapter linking these to themes in *Moses and Monotheism*. In addition, the aim of this initial chapter is to introduce the reader to the main themes and "characters" in this story who occupy and enliven the narrative of Freud's thought-provoking book.

Moses and Monotheism, Freud's last book, is a fascinating, controversial, quirky and ultimately a thought-provoking work that challenges the reader to step outside one's long-held beliefs and consider alternate points of view. Was Moses, who saw the face of God and received the Ten Commandments, originally an Egyptian? And perhaps an enraged Moses did not destroy those tablets, but instead quieted his fury against the Israelites worshipping the Golden Calf while protecting those laws? Furthermore, perhaps it was not Moses who crafted the concept of one God, but rather he had borrowed that idea from a heretic Pharaoh, Akhenaten, which then became the core of Judaism? And what is the connection between Moses and the source of the centuries' old anti-Semitism? These queries have a cumulative effect on the reader who may find himself/herself somewhat disoriented, but with Freud as our Virgil we arrive at understanding his arguments though we may not agree with his conclusions.

DOI: 10.4324/9781003272045-1

Why Did Freud Write *Moses and Monotheism*?

Moses and Monotheism was the culmination of Freud's attempt to understand several interdigitated themes that impacted him during his later life; however, we must be cautious and follow Chasseguet-Smirgel's (1988) advice which encouraged prudence in trying to understand Freud's motives when she states, "I consider that we have not yet discovered all the intentions of Freud's *Moses*" (p. 260). One unmistakable tributary was the rise of Nazism and the accompanying anti-Jewish laws in Germany which began in 1933 with the burning of books by Jewish authors, including those by Freud, as Hitler took power; slowly, at first not to alarm the general public, but then with a growing ferocity the Jewish population was cruelly marginalized by the anti-Jewish decrees. It is no coincidence that Freud began writing *Moses and Monotheism* a year later in 1934. This gradual nightmare was frighteningly captured in the enduring words of the Lutheran pastor Martin Niemoller:

> First they came for the socialists, and I did not speak out –
> Because I was not a socialist.
> Then they came for the trade unionists, and I did not speak out –
> Because I was not a trade unionist.
> Then they came for the Jews, and I did not speak out –
> Because I was not a Jew.
> Then they came for me – and there was no one left to speak for me.

Freud was then in his late seventies and accurately sensed the immense threat that Hitler's legions were to his way of life, his beloved Vienna and to psychoanalysis when his books were burned in Germany. Freud considered himself a German who happened to be Jewish, but he was well aware of the anti-Semitic history which plagued his people over the centuries:

> I have reason to believe that my father's family were settled for a long time on the Rhine, that, as a result of persecution of the Jews during the 14th or 15th century, they fled eastwards… into German Austria.
> (1925, p. 8)

Freud was mortified by Hitler's growing bellicosity during the 1930s and he struggled against the recognition that remaining in Austria was increasingly dangerous for him and his family, that like his father's family four centuries earlier, he, too, would have to flee persecution. As the decade rolled on, Freud was horrified as the Nazis grew more resolute in ostracizing the Jews with passage of the 1935 Nuremberg Laws which excluded them from citizenship and deprived them of basic rights. In addition, Freud faced another painful challenge from which he could not escape – the cancer of his jaw and the numerous surgeries he suffered which plagued him throughout the decade. Perhaps his worst suffering was in 1935 when Freud endured the most excruciating of these surgeries, from which he barely survived. It seems likely that the unrelenting Nazi degradations of his homeland and people combined with his physical pain to create a different kind of agony: "Why do people hate the Jews?" It is this question, more than any other, that authors consider as Freud's primary motive for writing *Moses and Monotheism*, an assertion that cannot be denied; however, his book also turns on another question, "Who are the Jewish people?" In response to this query, Freud offers us a unique version of a people who, once enslaved, are rescued from their bondage by a powerful leader; a man said to be born a Jew but perhaps he is actually an Egyptian nobleman?

Though the subtext of this book may deal with the questions such as "Why do people hate the Jews?" and "Who are the Jewish people?," we would be mistaken to consider *Moses and Monotheism* as a "Jewish book." To the contrary, there are many themes in this manuscript with contemporary relevance: the deep and long-lasting effects of slavery on a people; the desire for freedom and the search for leadership; considerations on the nature of religion and the origins of monotheism; the intergenerational transmission of trauma, and the lessons of unchecked hatred whether in the Holocaust, the current war in the Ukraine, or other instances of carnage too numerous to mention.

Freud began writing *Moses and Monotheism* in 1934 in Vienna and completed it in London in 1939. However, there is some evidence (Rolnik, this volume) that as early as 1925 he had postulated a thesis that Moses was actually an Egyptian who was killed by the angry Israelites. His formulation of the book and writing it occurred simultaneously with the Nazi rise in Germany and its later metastasis into Austria. The book was his constant companion during those years, and it is my belief that this writing brought him a sense of mastery and comfort during those horrific times of the dual terror that pained him so deeply: the growth of Nazism[1] and his fight with cancer of the jaw. In a similar way, but much less profound, editing this book has served an analogous purpose for me: the nightmare of the Covid virus, the one million American deaths which followed from its negligent and gross mishandling and ultimately reaching its seditious apex with the vicious attack on Congress by Trump's minions on January 6, 2021. I felt identified with Freud as he wrote about his work on what he called, "my Moses," as though his project was a solace in those bleak days. Similarly, beginning to edit this volume while watching the United States seemingly slide toward chaos and authoritarianism strengthened my identification with Freud: now I, too, had *my* Moses.

To a certain extent, every psychoanalyst identifies with Freud and in this opening chapter I examine *his* identifications as these relate to *Moses and Monotheism*. It is well known that he strongly identified with the biblical Moses and was fascinated by this historical figure[2] from his early years onward. Furthermore, given Freud's assertion that the idea of monotheism was originally developed by the heretic Pharaoh Akhenaten in the fourteenth century BC and subsequently adopted by Moses' pronouncements of Judaism, I think that Freud may also have identified with the iconoclastic Pharaoh as an originator of creatively new ideas – psychoanalysis and monotheism – that were disruptive of the status quo. I begin by tracing the development of Freud's identification with Moses from his childhood through to the end of his life and then move to a consideration of his claim that Akhenaten's revolution was the source of Moses' monotheism.

Freud's Identification with Moses

In a letter to Arnold Zweig (Letter to Arnold Zweig, 6/11/1934) Freud revealed a new work that he had undertaken and that "I have been writing something, and against my original intention it so took hold of me that everything else was put aside" and he also confided to Zweig that the question of Moses "has pursued me my whole life… [and that] Moses entirely engrossed his thoughts" (ibid., p. 194). Clearly, there was something about the Moses theme that resonated deeply in Freud's psychology which he could not resist. Later, in 1938, as he was hoping to obtain permission from the Nazis to emigrate to England, Freud wrote to Anna that "I also work for an hour a day at my Moses, which torments me like a 'ghost not laid'" (Jones, 1957, Vol. 3, p. 225). It is interesting that Freud, a lifelong atheist, would have been so taken with Moses, but his interest was with the *person* of the Prophet; thus, the original title of this work was *The Man Moses, an historical novel*. Yerushalmi (1991) offers the convincing notion that "the book can be read as a final chapter in Freud's lifelong case history" (p. 2).

When did this deep interest and identification with Moses arise in Freud? His *Autobiographical Study* (1925) begins with the brief statement that "my parents were Jews, and I have remained a Jew myself" (p. 7). I will not go into great detail regarding his family and its dynamics but will discuss aspects of his childhood and early years that are relevant to his affection for Moses. His great-grandfather and grandfather were called "Rabbi," though it was not certain whether they were truly rabbis since the term was often a title of respect (Jones, 1953, Vol. 1). His parents were genuinely supportive of their son: his father fostered the young man's intellect and they shared a good sense of humor as well as a similar physique. Furthermore, as his mother's first born of eight children, he was the recipient of her sole attention, who referred to him as "mein *goldener Sigi.*" As Jones commented, "a man who has been the indisputable favorite of his mother keeps for life the feeling of the conqueror, the confidence of success that often induces real success" (ibid., p. 5).

Freud's family was secular and, like many assimilated families, celebrated Passover each year with the ritual Seder that memorialized Moses' heroic role in the Exodus from Egypt. Freud began reading the Old Testament when he was seven years old and manifested a "deep engrossment in the Bible story" (Yerushalmi, p. 77), an interest that Ernest Jones attributed to the beautiful illustrations and woodcuts of the family's Philippson Bible. Anzieu (1986) highlights that

> the book opened up unknown territories for the young boy… [including] pictures that revealed bird headed Egyptian gods, the early history of God's chosen people, the Jews, Moses' Tables of the Law…
>
> (p. 17)

These discoveries surely fired up the young Freud's imagination and it does not seem too far-fetched to imagine a seven-year-old boy being drawn to the mighty and heroic figure of Moses who single-handedly (and with the help of God) delivered his people out of hundreds of years of bondage in Egypt, commanding with his powerful staff the parting of the Red Sea, and defeating through his guile the Pharaoh's chariots. This is the stuff of latency age fantasy with which a youngster might readily identify. Jones also describes Freud's youthful fascination with heroic leaders, including Alexander the Great (Anzieu, 1986), after whom he suggested to his parents that the youngest sibling, Alexander, be named.

But his greatest hero worship was saved for Hannibal who, with his armies of men and elephants, crossed the Alps in order to conquer Rome in the Second Punic war (218–201 BC), a daring invasion challenged by the opposing Roman forces and the elements; depicted in Turner's (1838) painting, *Hannibal Crossing the Alps*,

> in which we see his troops overpowered by, and cowering before, the charcoal stormy skies and the lashing of snow. The blackness of the storm appears like a huge mouth about to devour the dispersed soldiers
>
> (Brown, 2019, p. 128)

According to Jones, Freud favored Hannibal, a Carthaginian, in the Punic Wars which, in his mind was payback to Rome for its destruction of the second Temple in Jerusalem in 70 AD. In addition, Freud acknowledged in *The Interpretation of Dreams* (1900) that Hannibal

> had been the favorite hero of my later school days... [and that] the figure of the Semitic general rose still higher in my esteem. To my youthful mind Hannibal and Rome symbolize the conflict between the tenacity of Jewry and the organization of the Catholic Church.
> (p. 627)

Another of his boyhood idols was André Messena (1758–1817), who rose from a very modest background without a formal education to a position of prominence, whom Napoleon called "the greatest name of my military empire." Like Hannibal, he was a swashbuckling figure: born 100 years before Freud, it is difficult to assess his interest in Messena, but perhaps that he was rumored to be Jewish was part of his mystique. I suspect that the story of a young Jewish man rising from a humble background to one of notoriety appealed to Freud: he was at the top of his class for seven years in the Gymnasium which earned him "special privileges"; yet, as he began University at 17 years old, he discovered that "I was expected to feel myself inferior and an alien because I was a Jew" (1925, p. 9). His refusal to accept a lower rank and succumb to the allegedly shameful status of a Jew was certainly strengthened early in his life through these identifications with both his parents, Hannibal, Messena, and other figures that bolstered his independence of thought. Perhaps these admired figures were later condensed to form a powerful internal identification in Freud's mind of Moses as a strong figure who stood up to the Egyptians?

Freud's relationship with the Catholic Church was ambivalent and he feared that his new book, which posited that Moses was actually an Egyptian, would further push his ambivalent relationship with the Church in a negative direction. Freud, recalling the earlier opprobrium against *Totem and Taboo*, worried that his version of Moses would be met with even more severe criticism and that he "would be risking the banning of analysis in Vienna and the cessation of all our publications" (Jones, Vol. 3, p. 193) by the Catholic Church. Paradoxically, he was mindful that as much as the Church could be critical of his work, it also provided a bastion of sorts because "only this Catholicism protects us against Naziism" (ibid., p. 194). Freud knew that in the eyes of the Roman Catholic hierarchy his assertion that Moses was an Egyptian amounted to a heretical claim in its challenge to the biblical story of Moses; thus, he rewrote parts of the book in order to mollify the clergy's reactions. Freud was, in effect, faced with juggling his version of Moses, keeping the Catholic hierarchy at bay and, perhaps most paramount of all, to keep psychoanalysis alive and safe from the Nazis.

Freud and the Statue of Moses

Freud traveled extensively in Europe and despite his fascination with the Eternal City he seemed to have had a neurotic inhibition to visiting Rome, a reluctance that lifted with the close of his four years of self-analysis (Cohen, 2012). It was through that self-analytic work that he was able to understand more fully his identification with an aspect of Moses: just as Moses was kept from entering the Holy Land because he disobeyed God, so Freud would be kept from his discoveries and that "he feared that the price of his triumph might be his own death" (Anzieu, p. 186). He had longed to see Michelangelo's famed statue of Moses, an inhibited desire that he had not permitted himself to satisfy despite the fact that "Freud's interest in Michelangelo's statue was of old standing," which Strachey noted in his Introduction to Freud's (1914) paper, "The Moses of Michelangelo." Finally, at the age of 45, Freud visited the sculpture during his first trip to Rome and stared at it as though communing with some unspoken secret of the figure and then in "a flash of intuition, and reflecting on Michelangelo's personality, they gave him [Freud] an understanding of it" (Jones, Vol. 2, p. 20). We do not know the content of what Freud concluded about Michelangelo's personality; however, this early first impression was the start of his speculations about the meaning of the Moses statue. Why did the sculpture affect Freud so deeply? Freud said "no piece of statuary has ever made a strong impression on me than this" (1914, p. 213). He was probably familiar with the statue since there was a plaster copy of it at the Vienna Academy of Art which he had surely seen on many occasions, but coming face-to-face with the-thing-itself was mesmerizing and he wrote to his wife that "I have come to understand the meaning of the statue by contemplating Michelangelo's intention" (translation from German by Jones, 1957); again, a vague comment that leaves us wondering where Freud's reflections led him.

Michelangelo's Moses (1513) is a momentous and beautiful achievement: located in the Basilica of San Pietro in Rome, this marble statue of Moses is nearly eight feet tall and depicts him seated in a throne-like chair, the two tablets of the Ten Commandments grasped by the fingers on his right hand and wedged between his right side and the chair. He has a long beard that appears braided and yet unruly, his left hand holding the bottom of the beard in his lap, and he is looking toward his left as though distracted by some activity. In his first interpretation of the sculpture, Freud notes the tension in the statue that conveyed

> feelings which in the next instant will launch his great frame into violent action. Michelangelo has chosen this last moment of hesitation, of calm before the storm, for his representation. In the next instant Moses will spring to his feet – his left foot is already raised from the ground

> – dash the Tables to the earth and let loose his rage upon his faithless people.
>
> (1914, p. 216)

This analysis of Moses looking in anger at the Israelites worshiping the Golden Calf and readying to destroy the tablets in his fury is the most frequent interpretation of Michelangelo's work of art. Upon returning home, Freud assiduously reviewed the numerous writings about the figure and seemed to slowly formulate his own theory about the Moses sculpture in his many subsequent visits to Rome over the years.

Freud's return to Rome in 1912 proved to be an important visit in his efforts to gain a more definitive perspective of the statue. He reported to Jones that he visited Moses every day and that Freud hired a sketch artist to draw detailed pictures of certain segments of the sculpture for him in order to inspect portions of the statue more closely. Ultimately, Freud concluded that the statue was not capturing the moment *before* Moses was about to rage at the idol worshiping Israelites and smash the Ten Commandments to the ground; rather, the sculpture depicted a different story. Noting that the biblical Moses was given to fits of rage, Freud asserted that the statue did not represent Moses about to lose control of his anger, but rather

> something new and more than human to the figure of Moses; so that the giant frame with its tremendous physical power becomes only a concrete expression of the *highest mental achievement* that is possible in a man, that of struggling successfully against the inward passion for the sake of the cause to which he has devoted himself.
>
> (p. 233) [italics added]

Freud here has adopted a perspective that others had not taken: that the statue captures the *endpoint* of a process in which Moses deployed "the highest mental achievement" of curtailing one's wrath and that the sculpture details Moses taking his seat in order to *preserve* the Ten Commandments rather than destroy them. This interpretation of Michelangelo's famous work seems to have evolved from Freud's original (1901) "flash of intuition" about the artist's intent and from his subsequent numerous visits to Rome.

Regarding his identification with Moses, Freud had been struggling with his own anger in 1914 when he wrote the paper about Michelangelo's sculpture and so his emphasis on the "highest mental achievement" of curtailing one's rage also applied to *his* personal struggles at this time: he had been "abandoned' by Adler, Rank, and, worst yet, by his protégé Jung, which stung him most since Freud had earlier considered him his most promising adherent. These losses surely tested Freud to restrain his anger and this theme likely colored his unique view of Moses curtailing *his* rage at the disloyal Israelites and preserving the Ten Commandments (i.e., psychoanalysis) from destruction. Interestingly, he returned from a trip to Rome feeling invigorated and wrote "The Moses of Michelangelo" (1914) in less than a week, but decided to publish it anonymously, against editorial advice from Rank and Sachs. He told his friend Karl Abraham that he viewed the paper as amateurish and would be an affront to Moses;[3] thus, it was published in *Imago* without an author's name, which was finally added in 1924 when the paper was published in his *Collected Writings*.

Three Heretics: Moses, Freud, and Akhenaten

Wilfred Bion (1970) has discussed the relationship between the *Establishment* and the *mystic/heretic*. The Establishment governs a group and maintains the continuity of a system, whether political, educational or otherwise, and that "One of its more controversial activities is to promulgate rules (known in religious activities as dogmas…)" (ibid., p. 73). With respect to psychoanalysis, Bion states the Establishment refers to "the ruling 'caste' in psychoanalytical institutes" which regularly require an infusion of new ideas from individuals we might call a "genius," "mystic," or "heretic." Given the subject of this discussion, I prefer the term "heretic," which implies a violent upheaval of the status quo. Bion notes that the heretic "is both creative and destructive" (ibid., p. 74) and

> The group and mystic/heretic are essential to each other; it is therefore important to consider how or why the group can destroy the mystic/heretic on whom his future depends and how or why the mystic may destroy the group.
>
> (p. 77)

Furthermore, Bion emphasizes the disruptive quality of the mystic/heretic which may produce creative developments in the Establishment; however, "the heretic can be destroyed and an attempt made to ensure the same fate for his ideas" (ibid., p. 112).

In *Moses and Monotheism* we are introduced to three liberators: Moses, Freud, and the Pharaoh Akhenaten (born Amenhotep IV): Moses unshackled the Israelites and led his people in an Exodus from their slavery in Egypt; similarly, Freud sought to free mankind from the oppression of neurosis, the imprisonment of the libido, and the fealty that religion often demands. The Pharaoh Akhenaten (1380–1353 BC) proposed a monotheistic religion to replace traditional Egyptian polytheism with the belief in one god, Aten, embodied as the disc of the sun. However, one man's freedom fighter may be another's heretic who disturbs the status quo and shakes the pillars of the establishment. Akhenaten, also known as the "heretic Pharaoh," is a mysterious and fascinating historical figure who, like Moses and Freud, upended the political and social milieu in which he lived and unleashed cultural reverberations that rippled throughout their societies for centuries to come. Akhenaten's bold break with Egyptian polytheism and institution of a radical new religion earned him the designation of "the first individual of human history" (Breasted, 1905). Yerushalmi (1991) considers Freud "the arch heretic of Judaism... [who brought about a] demolition of the biblical view of history... in which Moses is, in effect, apotheosized and takes the place of God" (p. 35).

The Pharaoh Akhenaten and his innovations in religion, culture, artistry, and architecture have been an object of fascination for many years since the mid to late nineteenth century and continue to capture the imagination. Like Bion's heretic, Akhenaten tore down the extant polytheism of Egypt and razed many of his father's impressive works, replacing these with new creations. However, as Bion has cautioned, Akhenaten's innovations proved in the end to be more destructive than creative. Freud's heresy was to upend many of our long-held beliefs and to offer shockingly new perspectives that jolted society on such matters as infantile sexuality, the importance of dreaming, the power of unconscious experience, to name a few. Freud, however, was concerned about the potential disruptive effects of his heretical theories and strove to minimize the unsettling effects on society of psychoanalysis; a stance he carefully managed in his relations with the Catholic Church, thereby diminishing the potential destructive elements of his "heresies."

Despite his deep interest in Egypt from childhood and his large collection of Egyptian statuary, it is interesting that Freud never wrote about Akhenaten until the last few years of his life in *Moses and Monotheism*. However, he encouraged Abraham to write a paper (1912) about the Pharoah, yet Freud never referred to his important colleague's article. What motivated Freud to pass this "assignment" to his valued colleague and friend, Karl Abraham, and perhaps there was something about this topic that he found troubling? At a dinner in Munich in 1912[4] which Freud and Jung attended, the after-dinner discussion was about Akhenaten who, according to Freud, had destroyed his father's polytheistic religion to create his own monotheism. In contrast, Jung disagreed and opined that the Pharoah was not motivated by his Oedipal jealousy, but rather that Akhenaten had engaged in an act of creativity. As Jung spoke, Freud, who had been listening intently, suddenly slipped off his chair in a faint and quietly fell to the floor. Jung, who was six foot two and massively built, picked up Freud, carried him to the lounge and laid him gently on the sofa.

However, Freud's faint was not the first in similar circumstances. In 1909, Freud and Jung were traveling to America to lecture at Clark University, in Worcester, Massachusetts.[5] In one of their casual conversations, Jung spoke avidly about the then newly discovered "peat bog" corpses, which were of anthropological significance. Freud fainted while listening to that discussion as well – and, on awakening, accused Jung of harboring death wishes toward him. Apparently, Freud's previous faint in Munich also arose from a suspicion that Jung wished him dead. It must have been humiliating to Freud to have been carried to the couch by his younger and stronger competitor and perhaps this episode was an unconscious enactment of Jung's "murder" of Freud just as Akhentaten demolished his father's polytheistic belief systems. And so charging Abraham to write about Akhenaten may well have saved Freud from having to face once more his embarrassment over the Jung encounters. Nevertheless, Abraham completed his essay about Akhenaten in early 1912 and it was subsequently published in the new journal, *Imago*. Freud responded quickly, saying "Just think of it, Amenhotep IV (Akhenaten) in the light of psychoanalysis. That is surely a great advance in orientation" (ibid., p. 112). Nearly a dozen years later, the discovery of Tutankhamen's tomb and its treasure led Freud (1923) to anticipate the eventual discovery of Akhenaten's burial site[6] and Abraham apparently suggested a trip to Egypt which Freud, now 67 years old, rejected because of his "limited vitality." Abraham (letter, 4/1/23) replied that "I will not have it that a trip to Egypt is quite out of the question for you," and he further urged him by telling his friend about a 75-year-old uncle of Abraham's who had recently traveled there, but Freud was not swayed.

Perhaps Freud's 'vitality' was not as diminished as he would have Abraham believe and that some anxieties were reawakened that inhibited him, just as he did not "allow" himself to visit Michelangelo's Moses until his mid-forties despite extensive travels in other regions? What Freud may have lacked in strength he surely made up for in his great determination and endurance. Battling cancer of the jaw and enduring many painful surgeries whilst the Nazis tormented him and his family, facing the arduous task of obtaining permission to emigrate to the United Kingdom, and deeply troubled that his creation, psychoanalysis, would be destroyed, having already been labeled "degenerate," Freud persevered for much of the last decade of his life, buoyed by his physician, family, friendships, and the ever-present company of "my Moses."

Notes

1 The Anschluss of Austria on March 11, 1938 preceded Freud's leaving Vienna on June 4, 1938, a harrowing three month period of Nazi torment of Freud and his family.

2 "Akhenaten is a figure of history without memory, Moses is a figure of memory without history," Assmann, J. (2014).

3 Jones asserts that Moses was a father figure to Freud; thus, Freud's assertion that the paper would be an affront to Moses is at the same time a disappointment to his internal father.

4 This was the last meeting of Freud and Jung.

5 Accompanied by Sandor Ferenczi.

6 Akhenaten's tomb has never been conclusively discovered.

References

Anzieu, D. (1986) *Freud's Self-Analysis*. NY: International Universities Press. (Original French publication, 1975).
Bion, W. (1970) *Attention and Interpretation*. London: Tavistock Books.
Breasted, J.H. (1905) *A History of Egypt*. London.
Brown, L. J. (2019) *Transformational Processes in Clinical Psychoanalysis: Dreaming, Emotions and the Present Moment*. Oxon, UK: Routledge.
Cohen, D. (2012) *The Escape of Sigmund Freud*. New York, NY: Overlook Press.
Chassguet-Smirgel, J. (1988) Some thoughts on Freud's attitude during the Nazi period. *Psa and Cont Thought*, 11: 249–265.
Freud, S. (1914) *The Moses of Michelangelo*. SE, 13: 211–238.
Freud, S. (1925) An autobiographical study. SE, 20: 8.
Freud, S. (1939) *Moses and Monotheism*. SE: 23: 3–137.
Freud, S. (1934) Letter to Arnold Zweig (6/11/1934).
Jones, E. (1957) *The Life and Work of Sigmund Freud, Vol.* 3. New York: Basic Books.
Turner, J. M. W. (1838) *Hannibal Crossing the Alps*.
Yerushalmi, Y. H. (1991) *Freud's Moses, Judaism Terminable and Interminable*. New Haven and London: Yale University Press.

Editor's Introduction to Chapter 1

Lawrence J. Brown

The publication of Freud's *Moses and Monotheism* in 1939 was met with considerable controversy from religious figures, historians, biblical scholars, and other academics. Eran Rolnik's chapter offers us a detailed account of the initial reactions to the book through the lens of one particular group, the members of the Palestine Psychoanalytic Society.[1] This was a deeply inquisitive and intellectually vibrant group which thought carefully and critically about Freud's often heretical stances in *Moses*.[2] His speculation that Moses was originally an Egyptian, and that monotheism, too, was an Egyptian creation, was seen by many as offensive and also dangerous because such claims would negate the very essence of Judaism, in effect, a bastardization of the religion. Rolnik immerses us in the lively and sometimes acerbic exchanges between the participants, some of whom wanted to "turn him into a kind of ancient prophet" and others seeing Freud as a turncoat against his own people. Another, Rabbi Chaim Bloch, asserted that Freud's "study of Moses and the Torah are abominable sacrifices to the anti-Semitic demon" (Bloch, 1950, p. 101).

Rolnik is also an historian who has masterfully captured the ambiance of these meetings and the liveliness of the exchanges between members. We see Freud on the defense, holding his ground against his detractors, but also receiving support from others for his claims. One of his associates wrote that it is concrete thinking to consider that Moses was an actual historical figure and then "it made no difference whether or not there actually was an ancient leader named Moses" (Rolnik, this volume), but what mattered was that Moses lives on in our psyches over the hundreds of generations as a great man internalized by his nation, whose teachings and laws unmistakably survive. Rolnik treats us to other encounters between Freud and his supporters and those who take issue with *Moses*, in particular Eitingon's tense relationship with the philosopher, Martin Buber. Rolnik's chapter is a lively introduction to the politics and disputes provoked by the publication of Freud's last book, *Moses and Monotheism*.

DOI: 10.4324/9781003272045-2

Notes

1 The Palestine Psychoanalytic Society was founded by Max Eitingon in 1933 and modeled on the Berlin psychoanalytic Polyclinic, also established by Eitingon. In 1948 it was renamed the Israel Psychoanalytic Society.
2 *Moses* will be used as a shorthand for the full title.

1 "The Jewish Offensive"

The Reception of Freud's *Moses and Monotheism* in Mandatory Jewish Palestine

Eran J. Rolnik

Freud has an assured place in the history of ideas and of science as a man of intellectual courage who turned his back on essentialist views of humanity and on the Darwinist, biologistic, and racist theories that reigned supreme in the psychiatric thinking of his time. He founded a science of subjectivity based on investigation of the unconscious dynamic but universal psychological mechanisms that lie behind human differences and mental diversity. Paradoxically, in the 1930s, just when the explosive political potential of ethno-psychological and neo-Lamarckian views became apparent, Freud once again took up the idea of the hereditary transmission of character traits, leaving his heirs an enigmatic legacy in the form of the eerie theory of Judaism that he offered in his book *Moses and Monotheism* (1939a). Few texts in his oeuvre have proved as enduringly controversial as the work in which he applied the psychoanalytic tools he had developed over 40 years to an examination of the iconographic representative of the Jewish ethos – Moses, the greatest of the prophets.

In my book *Freud in Zion: Psychoanalysis and the Making of Modern Jewish Identity* (Rolnik, 2012), I searched for the mental and historical conditions under which the reception of Freud's teachings and the practice of psychoanalysis as therapy became possible in Jewish Palestine/Israel during the first half of the twentieth century. My study hypothesized and laid out the particular set of cultural and historical conditions, hopes, and anxieties which made it possible for psychoanalysis to emigrate from Central Europe and flourish in the *Yishuv* – the Jewish society of Palestine under British mandate.

In engaging with Darwinism, Nietzscheism, socialism, existentialism, and psychoanalysis, Zionist thinking ranged far and wide across the field of modern science and philosophy. These intellectual movements played an important role in the process of secularization that European Jewish society underwent, and provided (sometimes incompatible) justifications, arguments, and values that were appropriated into the Zionist movement's variegated ideological arsenal. Works by Darwin, Marx, Nietzsche, Spinoza, and Freud were widely discussed and debated within the Jewish

DOI: 10.4324/9781003272045-3

community as Zionism was beginning to shape the discourse on the political legitimation of this community and its self-understanding.

Zionist discourse deemed especially important those scholarly works that could offer alternatives to the traditional religious explanations for the existential plight of the Jewish people. Translations of Freud's essays into Hebrew were only second to those of Theodore Herzl and Max Nordau in the four decades that preceded the establishment of the Jewish state. Many of Freud's critics in Jewish Palestine had a penchant for speculating on the relationship between the Jewish origins of the creator of psychoanalysis and his theories. Some even went so far as to claim that his concept of repression should be viewed as an acknowledgment of his faith. The local debate over the Moses essay conflated a number of debates of historical significance. It could therefore be regarded as a particular case study for an interpretive community debating a new Freudian text; without hindsight, refracted through differing historical, ethical, and ideological sensibilities.

The members of the committee that in 1942 awarded the Tchernikovsky translation prize to the Odessa-born Zvi Wislavsky for his Hebrew rendering of *The Psychopathology of Everyday Life* emphasized that the excellence of his translation of Freud's book lay in its use of the language of the Mishnah and midrash, creating an illusion that "one of our ancients" wrote the original.[1] The committee's statement displayed the prevailing tendency of local *intelligenzia* to view Freud's theory as a manifestation of his Jewish origin (Rolnik, 2012). The desire to impart Freud's teaching to Hebrew-language readers in a prophetic-biblical style, and to turn him into a kind of ancient prophet, reached its climax during the 1940s, a formative period for Hebrew culture. The purpose was to make Freud's works part of the Hebrew literary canon, rather than something created outside it. True, since the publication of *Moses and Monotheism*, Freud's works were read eagerly but were not given easy acceptance, even after being "converted" by their translators. In fact, to Hebrew readers, it seemed that the doctor from Vienna who coined the term "repression" had already given away, in *The Psychopathology of Everyday Life*, his neurosis regarding his Jewish descent. When the translation came out, the poet Shin Shalom (Shalom Yosef Shapira) published an angry article with the headline "Freud's repressed Judaism." Shalom wrote of Freud's "repressed fundamental experience," manifested in his theory of self-disclosure and confession. He described how he himself broke free of the "initial intoxication" he had felt upon making an acquaintance with Freud's theory, which gave the concept of repression a central place. Shalom related that he had eventually reached the conclusion that he had to judge Freud according to his own standards. Was it just a coincidence that the creator of psychoanalysis was a Viennese Jew of the generation of assimilation, who hoped to find a solution for his own ills in the obliteration of his Jewish self? Shalom had no doubt that the repressed Judaism of Freud and his generation was the root experience behind his theory:

> The generational cry of the anguished Jewish nation that was compelled to repress and conceal its birth and its explicit name, its desire and its mission, in order to give in to the forceful ruling gentile reality of the world and all that is in it is what gave rise to the crushing and broad wings of this theory. Herzl, a member of Freud's generation and a party to his fate at first, was in fact the great discoverer and great redeemer of that depressed fundamental experience that Freud himself, originator of the theory of repression, could not comprehend. (Shalom, 1942, p. 318)

Herzl and Freud, each in his own way, were products of the repression experienced by the Jewish people. But while the former emancipated the Jews from being ruled by gentiles, Shalom maintained, Freud's theory was an expression of the way in which the Jews repressed their true desires. In Freud's text Shalom found the tragedy of the Jews of the West and of the entire Diaspora, which "is compelled to repress its connection to itself, to fear both the priest and the warrior … and to cast the newborn son into the Nile."

Shin Shalom's angry tirade about Freud's repressed Judaism was written at the height of the Second World War, at a time when many of the Yishuv's leaders and intellectuals found it difficult to shed their ambivalent attitude toward the Jewish immigrants from Central Europe. They felt a need to leaven their display of empathy and solidarity with no small amount of condemnation for the extent to which German-speaking Jews had assimilated into German cultural life. But the watershed in the way the Yishuv's intellectual circles of the 1930s and 1940s related to Freud was the latter's last great work, *Moses and Monotheism*, a volume that seemed to be aimed at reminding Freud's Jewish readership that the intellectual horizons of the originator of psychoanalysis, and the pressing needs of his fellow Jews, whether Zionist or non-Zionist, could never sit well together.

Impossible Confession

From the moment of its publication, Freud's book on Moses has taken its readers – analysts and non-analysts alike – by surprise. It addresses the psychology of religion and biblical criticism. It is also a novel that rewrites a myth, a historical work on the emergence of the psychoanalytic idea, a monograph on the origin of neurosis in the individual and in society, as well as a political manifesto and a metaphorical biography. Noting all these elements in *Moses and Monotheism*, Ilse Grubrich-Simitis (1997) termed it a "daydream." Edward Said (2003), for his part, aptly characterized the book with a musicological term, calling it a *Spätwerk*, a late composition, the kind that the composer leaves incomplete and which he writes largely for himself, leaving incompatible elements as they are – temporal, fragmentary, unpolished. Interesting testimony that has not yet been cited in the large body of work on Freud's Moses' essay can be found in an article published in 1950 in a Hebrew journal by Chaim Bloch (Blach), who studied Hasidism and kabbalah.[2] Bloch reported a meeting with Freud 25 years earlier at which they discussed Moses's origin and what might happen should Freud publish his thoughts on the matter:

> Twenty-five years ago I told Sigmund Freud, the eminent scholar, that his study of Moses and the Torah are abominable sacrifices to the anti-Semitic demon. I pleaded with him not to mow down what he had already planted, that the life of the Jewish people depended on him, and I warned him that the end would be that our people's enemies would place him among the traitors and informers.
>
> (Bloch, 1950, p. 101)

This was Bloch's opening to an account of his two encounters with Freud, during which Freud initially expressed his willingness to write an introduction to a book Bloch had written. But the first meeting ended in a major altercation, with Freud stalking out of the room in anger. Their conversation had turned to Judaism and Hasidism, Freud impressing Bloch with his knowledge. The former then produced two typewritten manuscripts and asked for his guest's opinion. "My heart went hollow and my hair stood up," Bloch recalled, "when I saw the headings 'Moses was an Egyptian born and bred,' 'Moses's Torah is the creation of Egyptian magi,' 'The Jews killed Moses,' no less. I read a few pages and my eyes filled with tears" (ibid., p. 102).

Bloch's account of his meeting with Freud around 1925 suggests that Freud already had in hand a manuscript that included the thesis that Moses was an Egyptian who was murdered by the Israelites. If true, this is evidence that *Moses and Monotheism*, the composition of which has always been dated to the years 1933–1938, was, in fact, written some time earlier. Bloch wrote that he told Freud that publication of the manuscript would be disastrous for the Jews, and Freud replied that "The truth causes neither a disaster nor danger." Bloch iterated that "Every man creates whatever truth he likes for himself and that there is no truth in the world as great as silence. The anti-Semites will lick their fingers when they read your studies." Freud responded that "he was repelled by the idea that we are chosen and superior to other nations," and held forth on his negative opinion of religion. To support his claims, he quoted from Theodor Herzl's Zionist novel *Altneuland*. He also cited the claim made by the writer Max Nordau, Herzl's partner in the founding of the Zionist movement, that the Holy Scriptures are a pile of superstitions and traditions from Egypt. Freud linked his manuscript with Nordau's writings:

> I will not deny that when I read [Nordau's] book on consensual lies and his sentence on the Holy Scriptures, I decided to take up this problem.

> After all, it cannot be claimed that Nordau harmed our nation! To the best of my knowledge the Jews admired Nordau when he was alive and honor his memory after his death. Nordau did not offer any proof of his statement that the Torah contains Egyptian traditions, but rather based his arguments on common sense alone. I have based my conclusions on evidence that no eye has yet seen.
>
> (ibid., p. 105)

At this point, the argument grew heated. Bloch claimed that Nordau had repudiated his statements about the Bible and had regretted allowing himself to be carried away by gentile biblical critics. Freud claimed that Nordau had never recanted. Bloch adduced evidence in support of his claim, a conversation Nordau had with Reuven Breinin, a Zionist journalist and critic, during which he acknowledged that he had been mistaken. Freud produced a letter he had received from Nordau in which the latter congratulated him for "your courage to uncover the truth about Moses and his Torah" and complained that the newspapers had spread a rumor that he had told Breinin he regretted what he had said about the Holy Scriptures. In the letter, Nordau denied the allegation categorically. Freud also showed Bloch the most recent edition of Nordau's book *The Conventional Lies of Our Civilization* (1913) to demonstrate to Bloch that its author had not revised his critical attitude toward the Bible. Bloch's transcription of the conversation indicates that the argument went on for quite some time. Bloch expressed his reservations, censured Freud, pleaded with him to file away his study of Moses – all to no avail. Freud even argued that his new findings were not based on vague ancient sources of the type cited by the Hebrew author Micha Josef Berdichevsky, but, rather, on new evidence that could not be denied.

Max Nordau's *The Conventional Lies of Our Civilization*, which condemns religion as a falsehood, was published in 1883 and was a great success (Gilman, 1993). The title does not appear in the bibliographies of Freud's works, nor was it in the library Freud brought to London. Yet, if we take Bloch's report at face value, Freud was acquainted not just with Nordau's book but also with Berdichevsky's writing on the subject. This is a new and interesting claim, especially in light of the fact that neither is cited anywhere in the writings of Freud published so far. Freud was almost certainly referring to Berdichevsky's great work *Sinai and Grizim*, in which he sought to prove that a critical reading of the Bible, Mishnah, Tannaitic, Talmudic, and rabbinic literature throughout the ages reveals an unending conflict between centers of power and spiritual leaders. It is hard to resist the temptation to speculate about why Freud chose not to cite Nordau's and Berdichevsky's studies in support of his ideas. The most obvious answer is that the writings of these two men were part of a scholarly discourse of a particularistic Jewish nature debated within the context of the Zionist movement. Citing them would have directed the debate over the figure of Moses from its innovative psychoanalytic context and restricted it to its traditional theological and historical aspects. Freud certainly must have known, however, that, in the final analysis, this strategy would not safeguard his book from a "Jewish offensive."

When Bloch saw that his claims had been countered, he tried another strategy. "'The measure that a man uses to evaluate others is used to evaluate him'," he told Freud, quoting a passage from the Mishnah. "Thousands of years from now some investigator will appear who will provide murky evidence that Prof. Sigmund Freud, originator of psychoanalytic science, was an Egyptian and his teachings are Egyptian, and the members of his generation killed him." Freud was not alarmed by the possibility that some future scholar might similarly conjecture that the founder of psychoanalysis, was not really Jewish. "And so what if they do?" he replied. "May it be – the principal thing is that my theory endure." Furthermore, in his earlier work *The Moses of Michaelangelo* (1914), it is already apparent that one thing that attracted Freud to the figure of the prophet and to identify with him was the fact that Moses reached the highest spiritual level within reach of humankind: the ability to set aside his personal emotions for the good of, and in the name of, the goal to which he had dedicated himself. Freud's equanimity induced Bloch to offer a less scholarly and more sarcastic rejoinder: "Have you also examined the list of births and deaths in Egypt so that you have unimpeachable evidence that Moses was of Egyptian extraction and that the Jews killed him?"

Freud felt the sting. "I won't write the introduction to your book and I don't want to see you again," he snapped and strode out of the room. Bloch was left in shock. When the two ran into each other on the street a few years later, Bloch was surprised to discover that Freud had forgotten the episode; neither did he even recall that they had ever met. He asked Bloch to remind him what their conversation had been about and why it had ended so badly. Bloch recounted the story and Freud recollected the conversation. "I remember your insolence, and I indeed don't want to see you again," he said, and walked off." (ibid., p. 107.)

Much of the literature on *Moses and Monotheism* mentions that a draft of the manuscript included a subtitle: "A Historical Novel." Freud's letters to Arnold Zweig and Max Eitingon show that the subtitle was Eitingon's suggestion, one of many he offered as "safety measures" intended to minimize the uproar that the book could be expected to set off among its Jewish readers:

> Since we live at a time so close in its spirit to the time of the Inquisition, it would be legitimate to take the same precautions taken in that time. Let's equip Moses with a subtitle that will appease its dangerous opponents, such as for example "A Historical–Psychological Novel." We know, after all, the amount of truth that novels conceal. One thing is certain – as opposed to Arnold Zweig's advice, I believe

> that publishing this work privately or anonymously will not provide sufficient protection. And another thing about which we can undoubtedly be certain: the work must come out in the framework of the [psychoanalytic] publishing house. … Still, the idea of publishing a book by you in Palestine, privately, is a wonderful and entertaining idea. Unfortunately, however, I must oppose the idea. It is simply not practical.
>
> (Eitingon to Freud, October 14, 1934, in Freud & Eitingon, 2004, p. 881)

Eitingon was apprehensive about how reaction to the book would affect the acceptance of psychoanalysis in the Yishuv. Rumors about Freud's plan to publish a book about Moses had already spread through Palestine's Jewish community. Yehuda Dvir-Dwosis, who had translated other works by Freud, wrote to him to ask: "In light of the great travails of the Jewish people in these times, has the time not come to answer the question with which you concluded the introduction to the Hebrew edition of your Introductory lectures on Psychoanalysis: What is it that makes me Jewish?" (Dvir-Dwosis to Freud, November 30, 1938: courtesy of Ora Rafael)

In his reply to Dvir-Dwosis, Freud dispersed some of the clouds of mystery that surrounded what he had written eight years previously:

> I have nothing to add or revise in what I wrote then. The mysterious sentence to which you refer relates to the question about the way in which our common tradition manifests itself in our psychic life – a complex problem of a purely psychological nature [...] My next book, about Moses and monotheism, will be issued at the beginning of the year in English and German. Of course its translation into the Holy Tongue will gratify me greatly. It is an extension of the subject discussed in Totem and Taboo, applied to the history of the Jewish religion. I ask that you take into account that the material in this work is particularly likely to offend Jewish sensibilities to the extent that these [sensibilities] are not interested in submitting themselves to the authority of science.
>
> (Freud to Dvir-Dwosis, December 2, 1938: AFM)

And, on June 28, 1938, Freud wrote to "Meister Arnold" (Zweig), arguably his favorite émigré interlocutor during the 1930s, who was living in Haifa: "Could you imagine that my arid essay could, even if it were to fall into the hands of a man whose heritage and education had made him into a believer, unsettle his faith?" (Freud & Zweig, 1970, p. 163).

The responses to *Moses and Monotheism* from intellectuals and psychoanalysts around the world spanned the spectrum. But the book clearly reverberated particularly strongly in the Yishuv years before it became a popular subject for debate in the historiography of psychoanalysis. The reactions came in the form of letters and critical articles written by scholars, personal letters from psychoanalysts to Freud, and a lively public debate carried out in the Hebrew press. There was even one public letter written by a citrus grower, which he published in the country's most important literary magazine. Yisrael Doryon, a Jerusalem-based writer and physician who was then working on a book on the Austrian philosopher Josef Popper-Lynkeus, immediately wrote to Freud to report that he had discovered an identical idea – that Moses was an Egyptian – in Lynkeus's book *The Fantasies of a Realist*. Freud related to Doryon that it was a great honor to discover that he owed his idea about Moses's Egyptian origins to Lynkeus. He was unable to tell Doryon with certainty "exactly how Popper-Lynkeus's Fantasies" had found its way into his work, but he reminded Doryon that the innovativeness of his book on Moses lay not in its conclusions, but in the way he reached them (Doryon to Freud, September 15, 1938; Freud to Doryon, October 7, 1938: FCLC).

Indeed, the matter of Moses's true identity is not central in the work. Its principal contribution lies in the role played by Moses in bringing the monotheistic doctrine to the Hebrews, and the way that that belief shaped Jewish identity through the mechanism of "inheritance of memory-traces of the experience of our ancestors, independently of direct communication and of the influence of education by the setting of an example"; the "assertion that the archaic heritage of human beings comprises not only dispositions but also subject-matter – memory-traces of the experience of earlier generations." Without using the term *Nachtraeglichkeit* explicitly in the Moses study, Freud used the historical riddle concerning the origins of Jewish monotheism in order to make a revolutionary link between the psychoanalytic clinic and the theory of history, individual and group psychology. The results, however tentative, are far reaching for both the theory of history and psychoanalysis. The development of Jewish monotheism over the generations is akin to the clinical course of traumatic neurosis over the life of an individual, where dual temporality of the trauma and the latency period are the crucial moments (Rolnik, 2001; Eickhoff, 2006). Equally sophisticated is the essay's contribution to the understanding of anti-Semitism as a trans-historical unconscious and overdetermined social phenomenon. Freud used the figure of Moses to iterate his claim that racial and intellectual differences, not Jewish religion and practices, stood between the Jews and their Christian environment. These differences kept the Jews distinct from all other nations in a way that does not permit complete integration, but only superficial cultural assimilation (Rolnik, 2016).

Why did Freud devote his final strength to a speculative thesis about the extraction of the leader of the Hebrews and the implications of Moses's life for the destiny of his people? One of the answers to this question can be provided by another Jewish thinker, perhaps not so well known to psychoanalytic readers, who also viewed Moses, in his 1912 essay, as a critical nexus of mythos and logos, rationalism and religious faith. In many ways, Freud's answer is surprisingly like that of Ahad Ha'am (Asher Ginzburg), the founder of spiritual Zionism. Both men maintained that religion and tradition should be examined scientifically in order to uncover the deepest levels of the human psyche's thinking, feeling, and imagination. If this is done consistently, without anti-religious prejudices, we will be able to uncover the depths of human truth that were, in ancient times, revealed to humankind as divine truth. Ahad Ha'am's essay on Moses, like Freud's work on the same figure, shows him at the peak of his creative powers.[3] It opens by making a distinction between archaeology and history. In his view, archaeology is the study of "material truth," the truth Freud sought in his book. But, wrote Ahad Ha'am, the biblical figure of Moses should not be seen as a "true" archaeological figure. In his view, it made no difference whether or not there actually was an ancient leader named Moses. The Moses of the Bible was a mythological figure who reflected the Jewish nation's ideal view of itself. The fact that he was not an archaeological figure did not in any way diminish the figure's tremendous influence. The prophet as portrayed in the people's imagination, fixed in the nation's collective consciousness, was more real than any archaeological figure. It shaped Jewish experience and its historical path:

> Surely it is obvious that the real great men of history, the men, that is, who have become forces in the life of humanity, are not actual, concrete persons who existed in a certain age. There is not a single great man in history of whom the popular fancy has not drawn a picture entirely different from the actual man; and it is this imaginary conception, created by the masses to suit their needs and their inclinations, that is the real great man, exerting an influence which abides in some cases for thousands of years – this, and not the concrete original who lived a brief period in the actual world, and was never seen by the masses in his true likeness.
>
> (Ahad Ha'am, 1912, p. 306)

The most salient characteristic of Moses, according to Ahad Ha'am, is that he is a "man of truth" and a "man of extremes." In other words, he is a person who saw life as it really is, who adhered to the path he believed in, and who rose above his selfish interests in order to realize his sublime values. The sublime validity of these values derives from their objectivity, the fact that they express a realistic and precise view of the world. Divine truth is simple, absolute, objective truth. It is not the truth of an individual, but, rather, the truth for everyone. Ahad Ha'am even provided a Freudian psychological explanation for Moses's experience of revelation at the burning bush. He argued that the voice Moses heard, the voice of God, was the voice of the national spirit that Moses bore in his heart from the time of his forgotten childhood, which was later, following his education in Pharaoh's palace, covered up and shunted aside in his adult life. This repressed memory suddenly surfaced in Moses's psyche in the wake of two incidents. The first was when he killed the Egyptian taskmaster he saw beating a Hebrew slave, and the second was when he encountered two Hebrews fighting each other. In the latter instance, when Moses told them to stop, one of them castigated Moses for murdering the Egyptian and trying to conceal his crime. As a result, Moses fled for his life. He tried to forget what had happened but did not succeed. His flight weighed on his conscience. But then came the most important event of all: he awakened from his "fainting fit [and] temporary loss of consciousness" and understood that he had fled not from his personal destiny but rather from that of his people (cf. Schweid, 1985). Clearly, the Moses of Ahad Ha'am epitomizes a post traumatic individual in the analytic sense of the word.

In the monologue with which he concludes his book *Freud's Moses: Judaism Terminable and Interminable* Yosef Hayim Yerushalmi (1991) wrote that the theory of Oedipal morality that Freud put in final form in his book on Moses is incontrovertible proof of Moses's "non-Jewish" origin. The interminable repetition of the repressed, Yerushalmi argued, is the precise opposite of the Jewish telos that looks to a specific future. Yerushalmi's sweeping conclusion was that Freud hoped that psychoanalysis would gradually become an alternative Jewish religion, devoid of all transcendental, metaphysical, and irrational components.

> I think that in your innermost heart you believed that psychoanalysis is itself a further, if not final, metamorphosed extension of Judaism, divested of its illusory religious forms, but retaining its essential monotheistic characteristics, at least as you understood and described them. In short, I think you believed that just as you are a godless Jew, psychoanalysis is a godless Judaism.
>
> (Yerushalmi, 1991)

Just as Freud's Egyptian Moses is the outsider who brings the Israelites the tidings of monotheism, Freud the Jew is the outsider who brings psychoanalysis to the world. More recently, in *On the Psychotheology of Everyday Life: Reflections on Freud and Rosenzweig* (2001), Eric Santner has taken a less radical approach to the psychoanalytic project, one that reconciles it with the philosophy of Franz Rosenzweig, a German–Jewish philosopher of the early twentieth century. Santner proposed that these two post-Nietzschean thinkers were classic representatives of secular theology. If there was any inherent Jewish dimension to psychoanalytic thinking, it was reducible to the concept that psychic healing is a type of Exodus from Egypt, in a more general way – it means giving up the national project and the search for a "home" (Santner, 2001).

Edward Said reached a similar conclusion in his essay *Freud and the Non-European* (2003). For Said, Moses became paradigmatic for the encounter with the Other, or, to use Said's post-colonial language, with the "non-European." Both Moses, the founder of Jewish self-awareness, and Freud, the founder of psychoanalysis, should, thus, be placed among those "non-Jewish Jews" (Deutscher, 1968) such as Spinoza, Marx, and Heine, who operated simultaneously from within and outside their Jewish identities. These writers not only stress the universal imperative within their self-conception as Jews, but also mark that intermediate space in which the concept of identity manifests itself in general. In their reading of Freud both Said and Santner countered the banal claim that Freud's search for his roots in a tribe that adopted Moses as a leader was no more than an expression of Freud's yearning to return to his and his parents' childhood home and to the Jewish tradition he had shed during his adult life. In so doing, both Said and Santner did, in my opinion, more justice then Yerushalmi to the Freudian outlook on the concept of identity and on the role that a psychoanalytically informed leadership can play in the formation of groups, nations and in politics in general. Freud's Jewish identity, like Moses's, was, a partial, broken identity that acknowledged that the psychology of the individual, like that of the collective, contains within it heterogeneous and fortuitous elements and identifications that have their source in influences lying outside consciousness and personal history. The paradox in the Freudian conception of identity derived from the inability of a whole and integrated identity to be achievable via a narcissistic search for the like, aided by the expulsion or evacuation of the different. Rather, the Jews elevated their capacity for abstract thinking and spirituality through the incorporation of the foreign, different, stressful, and unpleasant within the boundaries of the self, or the group. If there is a lesson to be learnt from the history of the Jews is that Identity is possible only if we mitigate the individual as well as the group's propensity for disavowal and acknowledge the presence of the foreign (or the Other) within its boundaries.

It follows that when Freud sarcastically declared that he intended to get at the truth behind Moses's "true identity," even if it meant undermining his people's "national interests," he might have thought that his Moses essay would not only shed light on the rise of anti-Semitism, but would also help mitigate a particular Jewish nationalist response to it: Zionism's solipsistic tendencies. That such tendencies existed was proved by the Yishuv's reaction to the book.

The Jewish Offensive

A few months after Freud received Dvir-Dwosis's letter, Max Eitingon (who founded the Palestine Psychoanalytic Society in 1934) reported to him that the Yishuv was awash with rumors about the content of his new book, and that he had gained opponents even though none of his critics had yet read it in its entirety. Shortly after the publication date, Eitingon met for the first time with Martin Buber, whom he considered one of the most influential critics of psychoanalysis on the Yishuv's intellectual scene. Following the meeting, he notified Freud that, while he thought he had got through his incisive conversation with the philosopher with his honor intact, there could be no doubt that psychoanalysis in Palestine had a determined nemesis in Buber. While Freud's assumptions about the etiology of the dream or on totemism were unacceptable to Buber, he saw no need to voice his views. But when it came to *Moses and Monotheism*, Buber informed Eitingon that he "could no longer remain silent," and that he intended to come out with a public statement condemning the book (letter dated February 16, 1939, in Freud & Eitingon, 2004, pp. 918–920). Buber and "his sanctimonious pronouncements" against the psychoanalytic theory of dreams did not cost Freud any sleep. "Moses is much more vulnerable and I am prepared for the Jewish offensive on it," he assured Eitingon (Freud to Eitingon, March 5, 1939, ibid., pp. 920–921). In 1945, when Buber published his own book on Moses, he rejected the approach of Bible scholars who cast doubt on the historicity of this Hebrew leader and wrote "that a scholar of so much importance in his own field as Sigmund Freud could permit himself to issue so unscientific a work, based upon groundless hypotheses, as his *Moses and Monotheism* (1939), is regrettable" (Buber, 1958, p. 7).

Eitingon himself had a hard time with *Moses and Monotheism*. Apparently, he read drafts of the manuscript prior to publication. His letter of thanks to Freud betrays the bewilderment of even Freud's most loyal admirers, especially his disciples in Palestine, over this work. Eitingon's ambivalence was evident between his lines of praise. He seems to have realized that the book could shut the door on his teaching psychoanalysis at the Hebrew University. Establishing a chair in psychoanalytic studies now seemed further away than ever.

> There is something exceptionally symbolic in the fact that your book on Moses arrived here on the Passover holiday, about which the Haggadah relates that God took the Jews out of Egypt "with a strong hand and an outstretched arm" [Eitingon wrote this phrase in the original Hebrew, but in German letters]. One can somehow sense the analogy in your book. Piercing logic, and a charm that cannot be withstood. That is how you bring the reader close to you in the final section, repeating for him the difficult arguments you make in Part II. It is a fine book.
>
> (Eitingon to Freud, April 11, 1939, in Freud & Eitingon, 2004, p. 923)

Two weeks later Eitingon informed Freud that "some excitement" was evident in the public's reaction to the book (letter dated April 30, 1939, ibid., pp. 924–925).

In May 1939, the Palestine Psychoanalytic Society convened a special meeting at which its members heard a lecture on the volume by Erich Gumbel, at the time Eitingon's senior candidate in training, who would soon become the Jerusalem Psychoanalytic Institute's first graduate (Gumbel to Freud, May 22, 1939: Archives of Freud Museum, London). The task of surveying this complex work was not an easy one. Even readers accustomed to reading Freud found that this book upset them. In his speech at this exceptional meeting, Eitingon intimated that the time might come when people would be skeptical of Freud's Jewish origins (Eitingon, 1950).

The Tel-Aviv based analyst Moshe Wulff (a former member of the analytic societies of Vienna, Russia and Berlin) was the first member of the Jerusalem Society to publish his impressions of the work. He noted that the book's structure and the wealth of subjects addressed made it much different from the rest of Freud's writings. While in his other books Freud had conveyed to his readers a feeling that he was totally on top of the subject at hand and that the main issues he faced as a writer were stylistic and aesthetic, in *Moses and Monotheism* Moses had "overwhelmed" Freud and suppressed his organizational and conceptual abilities. "I must acknowledge," Wulff wrote, "that I have never been so profoundly affected by a work of Freud's as I have been by this one." And Wulff ended his paper with a discussion of the "eternal question" of truth: "And so Freud called his book the 'Moses Novel.' Such things do occur in novels and in art: the Whole may even be fictitious, invented, the fruit of phantasy from top to bottom, yet it nevertheless remains the highest and most profound truth, an inner truth of the human soul" (Wulff, 1950, pp. 124–142).

The Hebrew press seethed and only with difficulty was able to provide space for all those who wanted to fulminate about the book. "Freud's war against Moses!" shouted a headline in the religious Zionist daily *Hatzofeh* (Kaminka, 1939). Moses defenders came from all walks of life: a citrus farmer, Nachum Perlman, was deeply affected by Freud's book. He sought to link his critique to the campaign then under way to persuade Jews to buy goods grown or manufactured in the Yishuv. Did the campaign, he queried, relate only to material items, or should not Jews also boycott intellectual and spiritual imports which undermine Jewish national interests? In an open letter to Freud published in the Yishuv's leading literary magazine, *Moznayyim*, headlined "Professor Freud and buying local," Perlman rebuked those who allowed themselves "to cast into the depths of the sea our spiritual possessions and, in spiritual matters, to open all gates wide to concepts entirely foreign to Judaism" (Perlman to Freud, July

2, 1939: AFM). Perlman did not simply write his open letter to Freud in Hebrew. He translated it into German and sent it directly to Freud, adding a covering letter:

> I presume to address you, sir, as I do below, despite being no more than a layman with regard to your scientific profession. I write from the point of view of a Jew who has lived in the Land of Israel for the last thirteen years, not by coincidence, but because he feels that the continued existence of the Jewish people is something valuable for all of humanity. But because I am, sir, as I have already said, no more than a layman, I do not permit myself to critique your book Moses but only to ask you one question. You must certainly know, sir, that at this time a large number of our brethren view the results of Biblical criticism as the actual content of the Jewish people's literature, without thinking through to themselves that in doing so they are cutting off the branch on which they sit, a thing that is on the one hand consistent, since it is known that we, the Jews, are "air people [...] But not only does the reading public welcome this science, so do intelligent people and well known Jewish writers among those who steer them, without considering the fact that all the archaeological excavations that have been conducted so far that contain any sort of indication regarding the Torah all confirm the words of the Bible and prove the flimsiness of Biblical criticism.
>
> (Perlman to Freud, July 2, 1939: Archives of the Freud Museum, London)

Was not affirmation or repudiation of Biblical criticism by Jews intended, whether they were aware of it or not, to justify their betrayal of the foundations of the Jewish religion and the Torah's commandments, Perlman asked Freud. He answered the question himself:

> I believe that you, Herr Professor, are the best man to offer a full answer to my question, and I believe that in answering this question you will have the privilege of doing more for Jewish existence than you did with your book Moses.
>
> (ibid.; the original letter is reproduced in Rolnik, 2010)

Raphael DaCosta of Jerusalem also wrote to Freud after reading the book. Unlike Perlman, he enjoyed it immensely. Nevertheless, he was of the opinion that the evidence Freud had adduced was insufficient. Freud based his claims on the thesis that the figure of Moses was actually composed of two different men, each of whom represented a distinct set of beliefs. This had to be the case, Freud maintained, because the differences between the two deities represented in the Torah are so huge that it would be difficult to conceive that they had been put forward by a single priest. DaCosta wrote that he would have accepted this proposition had it not implied that the Israelites had chosen the wrathful Egyptian priest. The other priest, the merciful man from Midian, was not appointed to represent Aton, the civilized sun god (DaCosta to Freud, April 23, 1939: AFM).

Freud took the reservations of this Jerusalem reader seriously, and seems even to have regretted his speculative proposal that the biblical Moses was actually a composite of two men, a "good" priest and a "bad" priest. He replied to DaCosta:

> There is indeed a difference in the natures of the two figures called Moses that I am unable to explain, but it could be said that the matter is not of great significance. We know very little about the second Moses, who is of course an invention of mine, and I could have made do without the comment about his even-temperedness.
>
> (Freud to DaCosta, May 2, 1939: AFM)

Another point DaCosta made to Freud concerned the implications the book should have for the Jewish view of the world. He asked Freud whether the two beliefs, in religious truth and in scientific truth, were mutually exclusive. In other words, is there a way to reconcile rationalism with faith? Would Freud permit his fellow Jews to maintain their theological truth along with material truth, or did he insist that historical truth, which he recreated in his psychoanalytic studies, replace religious truth?

In *The Future of an Illusion* (1927), Freud had already taken a firm position on the order of precedence of varying truths. He claimed that religious thinking of all kinds was simply the civilized incarnation of infantile sexuality, and that religion was tantamount to a neurosis that needed to be overcome. Freud repeats this position in *Civilization and Its Discontents* (1930). But Freud's work on Moses seems to have led him to a somewhat more nuanced view, implying a certain revision of his conception of religious faith. In *Moses and Monotheism,* he acknowledged two truths, one religious and subjective, and the other archaeological and objective. He did not present these as contradictory, but rather as complementary two positions that a person can move between. In the newer work, Freud gave historical truth itself the special status of being able to include several truths. It did not derive from an unambiguous rational decision of any type, but, rather, from an ongoing process of give and take that also allowed phantasmic, mythological, and subjective elements to play a role in a dynamic representation of reality. The grafting of religious and historical truth to each other (in the absence of the ability to recreate lost material truth in the positivist sense) constituted one of the most important goals of the psychoanalytic project. The ability to tolerate doubt did not deprive Freud of the right to feel that he was persuaded of the truth of his conclusions. Freud repeatedly addressed the question of certainty vs. skepticism throughout *Moses and Monotheism*, and, in doing so, re-enacted and demonstrated for his readers the convoluted nature of psychoanalytic epistemology. As Blass (2003) has pointed out, hoovering between conviction and doubt, Freud's Moses, and in particular his employment of the Puzzle metaphor in the text, is a contribution to psychoanalytic epistemology and clinical theory. It is in this later work of his that Freud gave final expression to the dialectic view of the concept of "truth" in its unique psychoanalytic form. He stressed the tentative and speculative nature of his account, but did not let this prevent him from recognizing that he was approaching the truth. Indeed, his reply to DaCosta shows that as soon as he reached conclusions about historical truth, he could not put in its place another truth simply because the latter was worth believing in from a religious point of view. Freud wrote to DaCosta:

> I am amazed at the way you succeed in bringing together the findings of scientific investigation and belief in the accuracy of the biblical account. I myself would be incapable of such acrobatics. But who gave you the right to grant the Bible a monopoly on the truth? All you are saying is that I believe because I believe.
>
> (Letter dated May 2, 1939: AFM)

The question, then, is what is the nature of that truth that Freud proclaims? He opens his book hesitantly, qualifying his assertions, but, as the book proceeds into the third and final part, he seems to become more and more certain of himself, until, by the end, he states his thesis unambiguously. Did Freud convince himself on purely scientific grounds, or was he asserting a belief? After all, the scholar must have no less faith in historical and scientific truth than the religious person has in biblical truth. Freud tried to resolve this paradox by skipping back and forth between two of his favorite genres, the historical novel and the clinical case study. It becomes clear to the reader that *Moses and Monotheism* is neither a positivist historical account nor speculative psychology. Rather, it is a readers' response text devoted to examining the theory of psychoanalytic epistemology and the persuasive force that the truth – whether about the identity of the Hebrew leader or about the true value of the autobiographical memory that emerges during psychoanalytic treatment – can elicit from the person who seeks it. Freud thought that the historical novel genre could enable him, even though he viewed himself neither as a historian nor as a novelist, to address the question of the identity of this biblical figure in accordance with the rules of the clinical case study, in which the act of reconstruction is accomplished through the integration of historical and clinical evidence into the subjective narrative. Freud's biography of Moses can, thus, be seen as the last case study left to us by the creator of psychoanalysis.

Concluding Remarks

"There is something ridiculous about an ancient nation," writes Israeli novelist A. B. Yehoshua, "that is still, after some 3,300 years, hammering so intensely and so obsessively at the enigma of its identity, tirelessly searching for more and more explanations, definitions and versions of it" (Yehoshua, 2005). Freud's explorations of the "true identity" of Moses, leader of the Jewish nation, address this very conundrum. Identity, Freud told us, whether historical or psychological, of an individual, a group or a nation, is the product of mixture and borrowing, and always includes splits and repressions. Freud's fractured Jewish identity could thus serve, if not as an example, then at least as a metaphor for the yawning abyss separating the ideal of pure identity that nurtured the Zionist project and the psychoanalytic project, born in the Diaspora. Unlike the Zionists, Freud never rejected the Jew of the Exile, and, unlike the socialists, he never rejected bourgeois life. He did not pretend to be designing a "new man" free from the constraints of frustration or guilt, much less a "new Jew." Ironically, in this sense, the philo-psychoanalysis of the Yishuv's immigrant society, despite its contradictions and paradoxes, testified to the immensity of anxieties, anguish, and doubts that were the lot of those who tied their personal redemption to reborn Jewish nationalism in the Land of Israel. Zionism, to put it simply, might not have agreed with Freud, but very badly needed him.

Notes

1 Prize committee discussions, not dated, and letter of Mayor Israel Rokach to Wislavsky, January 29, 1945 (Tel Aviv City Archives). Max Eitingon wrote the introduction to the Hebrew translation.

2 Rabbi Chaim Bloch (Blach) emigrated from Galicia to Vienna in 1915. There he published extensively on Jewish legends and became known for his interviews and correspondence with famous Jewish scholars. In 1938, he immigrated to New York, and became known for his essays against Zionism.

3 Freud knew Ahad Haam personally (see Rolnik, 2012).

References

Ahad Ha'am (1912). *Selected Essays of Ahad Ha-'Am*, L. Simon (Ed.). Philadelphia: Jewish Publication Society [reprinted New York: Atheneum, 1970].

Blass, R. (2003). The puzzle of Freud's puzzle analogy: reviving a struggle with doubt and conviction in Freud's Moses and Monotheism. *International Journal of Psychoanalysis*, 84: 669–682.

Bloch, H. (1950). Recollections of my meeting and debating with Freud over Moses. *Bitsaron*, XXIII: 101–108 [Hebrew].

Buber, M. (1958). *Moses: The Revelation and the Covenant*. New York: Harper.

Deutscher, I. (1968). *The Non-Jewish Jew and Other Essays*. New York: Hill and Wang.

Eickhoff, F. (2006). Nachträglichkeit from the perspective of the phylogenetic factor in Freud's "Moses and Monotheism." *Scand. Psychoanal. Rev.*, 29(1): 53–59.
Freud, S. (1914) *The Moses of Michelangelo*. S.E., 13: 211–238.
Freud, S. (1927). *The Future of an Illusion*. S.E., 21: 3–56. London: Hogarth.
Freud, S. (1939a). *Moses and Monotheism*. S.E., 23: 3–137. London: Hogarth.
Freud, S., & Zweig, A. (1970). *The Letters of Sigmund Freud and Arnold Zweig* ,E. L. Freud (Ed.). London: Hogarth Press and the Institute of Psycho-Analysis.
Freud, S., & Eitingon, M. (2004). *Sigmund Freud–Max Eitingon Briefwechsel, 1906–1939*, M. Schröter (Ed.),Tübingen: edition diskord.
Gilman, S. (1993). Max Nordau, Sigmund Freud, and the question of conversion. *Southern Humanities Review*, XXVII(1): 1–25.
Grubrich-Simitis, I. (1997). *Early Freud and Late Freud: Reading Anew Studies on Hysteria and Moses and Monotheism*. London: Routledge.
Kaminka (1939) "Freud's war against Moses!" *Hatzofeh*, 17 August 1939.
Nordau, M. (1913). *Die conventionellen Lügen der Kulturmenschheit*. Leipzig: Elicher.
Rolnik, E. J. (2001). Between memory and desire: from history to psychoanalysis and back. *Psychoanalysis and History*, 3: 129–151.
Rolnik, E. J. (2010). Therapy and ideology: psychoanalysis and its vicissitudes in pre-state Israel (including some hitherto unpublished letters by Sigmund Freud and Albert Einstein). *Science in Context*, 23(4): 473–506.
Rolnik, E. J. (2012). *Freud in Zion: Psychoanalysis and the Making of Modern Jewish Identity*. London: Karnac.
Rolnik, E. J. (2016). "The bad, the mad and the functional – one antisemitism or many." Conference paper at the EPF Annual Meeting, Berlin 2016. www.epf-fep.eu/eng/article/the-bad-the-mad-and-the-functional-one-anti-semitism-or-many
Said, E. (2003). *Freud and the Non-European*. London: Verso.
Santner, E. (2001). *On the Psychotheology of Everyday Life: Reflections on Freud and Rosenzweig*. Chicago, IL: University of Chicago Press.
Schweid, E. (1985). *The Land of Israel: National Home or Land of Destiny*. Rutherford, NJ: Fairleigh Dickinson University Press.
Shalom, Y. S. (1942). Freud's repressed Judaism. *Moznaim*, 14: 317–319 [Hebrew].
Wulff, M. (1950). An appreciation of Freud's "Moses and Monotheism." In: M. Wulff (Ed.), *Max Eitingon: In Memoriam* (pp. 141–150). Jerusalem: Israel Psychoanalytic Society.
Yehoshua, A. B. (2005). An attempt to comprehend the infrastructure of anti-semitism [Hebrew]. *Alpayyim*, 28: 11–30.
Yerushalmi, Y. H. (1991). *Freud's Moses: Judaism Terminable and Interminable*. New Haven, CT: Yale University Press.

Editor's Introduction to Chapter 2

Lawrence J. Brown

The controversial topic of inherited memories from our repressed archaic heritages appears throughout *Moses and Monotheism* and in this chapter Peter Hoffer introduces us to Freud's thinking about this subject. He begins in 1983 with the German psychoanalyst, Ilse Grubrich-Simitis, who fortuitously discovered a paper written by Freud (1915), entitled "Overview of the Transference Neuroses,"[1] in a trunk of Ferenczi's papers. In the article, Freud offered a new theory about the origins of various mental illnesses, linking the sources of various psychiatric disorders to "inherited dispositions" from specific stages in human development. For example, Freud connected most anxiety related problems to "the influence of the privations that the encroaching Ice Age imposed upon [mankind, which] has become generally *anxious*" (1915, 13f.). Analogously, the putative origins of obsessional neurosis are traced to a somewhat later time in our prehistory in which the formation of the "primal horde" predominated. These primeval anxieties and fears join with heredity and everyday experiential factors in the creation of neuroses. This Phylogenetic Fantasy was not meant to replace standard psychoanalytic thinking about the development of neurotic and psychotic pathology, but rather added another dimension:

> The stages of development primal to civilized man are repeated, at least figuratively, in the mental development of the child up to adulthood.
>
> (Sterba, 1937, p. 27)

But perhaps even more radical than Freud's notion about the repetition of archaic themes was his

> assertion that the archaic heritage of human beings comprises not only dispositions but also subject matter – *memory traces of the experience of earlier generations.*
>
> (Freud, 1939, p. 99; italics added)

DOI: 10.4324/9781003272045-4

His claim that 'memory traces' from the primordial history of human beings live on in our psyches and become re-enlivened in times of trauma is perhaps the most objectionable assertion in *Moses and Monotheism*; however, Freud remained recalcitrant in holding to this Lamarckian belief of the inheritance of acquired characteristics. Regarding Freud's assertion that Moses was murdered by the Israelites, a crime that was subsequently repressed, Hoffer notes:

> In the case of Moses the principal traumatic event was his murder at the hands of his followers, which was subjected to the forces of repression for several generations, only to reemerge in the distorted form, condensed with the experiences of the groups that followed, who would coalesce into the cultural and historical nucleus of the Jewish people.

These concepts – the Phylogenetic Fantasy, the reappearance of 'repressed' memories from our archaic histories, the murder of Moses and the re-emergence of its memory after centuries of repression – are often challenging to wrap one's mind around and we are thankful to Dr. Peter Hoffer for the clarity of his writing and thinking.

Note

1 This paper has subsequently come to be known as the "Phylogenetic Fantasy." Dr. Hoffer's chapter discusses this in greater detail.

2 Freud's "Phylogenetic Fantasy" and His Construction of the Historical Moses

Peter T. Hoffer

On July 28, 1915, Freud wrote to Ferenczi:

> I am sending you herewith the draft of the XII [paper], which will certainly interest you. You can throw it away or keep it. The fair copy follows it, sentence for sentence, deviating from it only slightly. Pages 21–23 have been added since your letter, which I had waited for. Fortunately, I had anticipated your excellent criticism.
>
> (Falzeder & Brabant, 1996, p. 73)

With these mildly self-effacing remarks, Freud signaled to his friend and colleague that he had completed a series of papers with the intended title *Zur Vorbereitung einer Metapsychologie* (Preliminaries to a Metapsychology), which was destined soon to become the most important advance in psychoanalytic theory since *The Interpretation of Dreams* and the *Three Essays on the Theory of Sexuality*. Unfortunately, for reasons that must remain the subject of speculation, Freud published only five of the 12 papers, "Instincts and their Vicissitudes" (1915c), "Repression" (1915d), "The Unconscious"(1915e), "A Metapsychological Supplement to the Theory of Dreams" (1917d), and "Mourning and Melancholia" (1917e); the remaining seven were lost, presumably destroyed by the author himself, save for the 12th, which was discovered serendipitously in 1983 in a trunk containing Ferenczi's papers by the German psychoanalyst Ilse Grubrich-Simitis. Titled *Übersicht der Übertragungsneurosen* (Overview of the Transference Neuroses), it was first published in German in 1985 by S. Fischer Verlag and in English translation in 1987 by Harvard University Press with the words "A Phylogenetic Fantasy" added to the original title. The addition stems from a remark by Freud himself in a letter to Ferenczi of July 18, 1915, to the effect that he "would like to have heard more critique about the phylogenetic fantasy" (Falzeder & Brabant, 1996, p. 68).

The critique from Ferenczi that Freud would have liked to hear more about referred to a letter that he had written six days earlier, in which he outlined the basis for "a series of chronological starting points in individual cases of illness, which runs as follows: Anxiety

DOI: 10.4324/9781003272045-5

hysteria – conversion hysteria – obsessional neurosis – dementia praecox – paranoia – melancholia-mania." (ibid., p. 66). The draft "Overview" begins with a detailed description of the six factors that form the distinguishing characteristics of the transference neuroses: repression, anticathexis, substitutive- and symptom formation, relation to the sexual function, and disposition, the first five of which had been introduced and elucidated to a large degree in the published metapsychology papers. This introductory section of the Overview is written in a telegraphic style, which makes it difficult to decipher.

When he comes to the sixth factor, however, Freud's style changes abruptly from a telegraphic into a more coherent narrative:

> Behind regression are hidden the problems of fixation and disposition. Regression, one can say in general, goes all the way back to a fixation point, in either ego or libido development, and it represents the disposition. This is thus the most decisive factor, the one that mediates the decision concerning the choice of neurosis.
>
> (1987 [1915], p. 9)

He continues:

> When the constitutional factor of fixation comes into consideration, acquisition [is] not eliminated thereby; it only moves into still earlier prehistory, because one can justifiably claim that the inherited dispositions are residues of the acquisition of our ancestors. With this one runs into the problem of the phylogenetic disposition behind the individual or ontogenetic, and should find no contradiction if the individual adds new dispositions from his own experience to his inherited disposition acquired on the basis of earlier experience.
>
> (ibid.)

With these matter-of-fact observations, Freud establishes the main thesis of the essay, that the three transference neuroses, anxiety hysteria, conversion hysteria, obsessional neurosis, along with the three narcissistic neuroses (called psychoses in today's terminology), dementia praecox, paranoia, melancholia-mania, have as their basis pathogenic factors stemming from lived experience in the developmental history of the individual, combined with inherited dispositions acquired in the prehistory of the human species. He then sets up a "phylogenetic series" premised on the assumption that the age of onset of each neurosis (that of anxiety hysteria being the earliest, melancholia-mania the latest), conforms to successive stages of human development during the Ice Age. Accordingly, anxiety hysteria and conversion hysteria, chronologically the earliest in the series, acquire their respective dispositions "under the influence of the privations that the encroaching Ice Age imposed upon [mankind, which] has become generally *anxious*" (pp. 13f.).

The disposition to obsessional neurosis and those to the narcissistic neuroses trace their origins to a later stage of prehistory, that which witnessed the formation of the "primal horde," which was the centerpiece for Freud's excursion into anthropology and the history of religion, *Totem and Taboo* (1912–1913). As the harsh conditions of the Ice Age gradually diminished, prehistoric man – in this instance the male of the species –

> learned how to investigate, how to understand the hostile world and how by means of inventions to secure his first mastery over it. ... Language was magic to him, his thoughts seemed omnipotent to him, he understood the world according to his ego. It is the time of the animistic world view and its magical trappings"
>
> (1987 [1915], p. 15).

These transformations formed the basis for the disposition to obsessional neurosis, in which

> [t]he overemphasis on thinking, the enormous energy that returns in the compulsion, the omnipotence of thoughts, the inclination to inviolable laws, are unchanged features.
>
> (p. 16)

At this point in his narrative, Freud departs from the topic of the transference neuroses contained in the title of the draft and launches into a discussion of the narcissistic neuroses, the dispositions to which are acquired by a "second generation" of prehistoric humans, which begins with the sons,

> to whom the jealous primal father does not allow full scope. We have indicated elsewhere [in *Totem and Taboo*] that he drives them out when they reach the age of puberty. [Psychoanalytic] experiences admonish us, however, to substitute another, more gruesome, solution – namely, that he robs them of their manhood – after which they are able to stay in the horde as harmless laborers. We may imagine the effect of castration in that primeval time as an extinguishing of the libido and a standstill in individual development. Such a state seems to be recapitulated by dementia praecox, which especially as hebephrenia leads to giving up every love object, degeneration of all sublimations, and return to auto-erotism.
>
> (p. 17)

In the next phase in the evolution of the primal horde,

> The threatened sons avoided castration by means of flight and, allied with one another, learned to take upon themselves the struggle for survival. This living together had to bring social feelings to the fore and could have been built upon homosexual satisfaction. …This phase of the condition … manifestly brings back paranoia; more correctly, paranoia defends itself against its return.
>
> (pp. 17f.)

The third and final phase of the evolutionary process creates the disposition to the last illness in Freud's phylogenetic series, melancholia-mania:

> If one looks at the characteristic alternation of depression and elation [in melancholia-mania], it is difficult not to recall the very similar succession of triumph and mourning that forms a regular component of religious festivities: mourning over the death of the god, triumphal joy over his resurrection. This religious ceremony, however, as we have surmised from the statements of ethnopsychology, only recapitulates in reverse the attitude of the brother clan after they have overpowered and killed the primal father; triumph over his death, then mourning over the fact that they all still revered him as a model … The mourning about the primal father proceeds from identification with him, and such identification we have established as the prerequisite for the melancholic mechanism.
>
> (pp. 18f.)

It is worthy of note that Freud made this last observation explicit in "Mourning and Melancholia" (1917e), which he completed before writing the present draft. It is equally noteworthy that in Freud's phylogenetic schema the dispositions to the transference neuroses are formed in earlier stages of prehistory than are the dispositions to the narcissistic neuroses and the changes in cultural development which evolve from them:

> If the dispositions to the three transference neuroses were acquired in the struggle with the exigencies of the Ice Age, then the fixations that underlie the narcissistic neuroses originate from the oppression by the father, who assumes, continues its role, as it were, against the second generation. As the first struggle leads to the patriarchal stage of civilization, the second leads to the social; but from both come the fixations which in their return after millennia become the disposition of the two groups of neuroses. Also in this sense neurosis is therefore a cultural acquisition."
>
> (1987 [1915], p. 19)

The operative words in the last sentence are "Also" and "cultural acquisition." In his brief summation of the draft "Overview," Freud leaves open the question as to what extent the ontogeny of modern neuroses (and psychoses) is dependent on both hereditary and experiential factors. What is certain is that both come into play. Mindful of the uncertainty regarding their origin and intensity in each individual, he closes his summation with a disclaimer:

> The parallel that has been sketched here may be no more than a playful comparison. The extent to which it may throw light on the still unsolved riddles of the neuroses should properly be left to further investigation, and illumination through new experiences.
>
> (ibid.)

Richard Sterba's *Dictionary of Psychoanalysis* (Sterba, 2013) originally published in 1937, contains an entry with the heading *Biogenetsches Grundgesetz* (biogenetic law). It reads:

> The biogenetic law states that ontogenesis is an abbreviated phylogenesis. That means that, in the course of the development of the germplasm to the mature individual, the stages of development of the species must be reiterated in abbreviated form. … Only with the advent of psychoanalysis has it been shown that the biogenetic law is also fully valid in the <u>psychic</u> sphere. The stages of development primal to civilised man are repeated, at least figuratively, in the mental development of the child up to adulthood. Not only are there numerous correspondences in the individual stages of mental development of the child with the psychology of primitive peoples and savages, which we consider to be remnants of earlier states of the cultural and psychic development of humankind, but the regressions of adults in <u>neurosis</u>, <u>psychosis</u>, and the <u>formation of groups</u> are also evinced by traits and peculiarities that we observe in primitive peoples.
>
> (pp. 27f. Emphasis in original)

The "biogenetic law," formulated by Ernst Haeckel (1868) in the late nineteenth century, was popularized in Freud's time by the phrase "Ontogeny recapitulates phylogeny." It has since been largely discredited by modern biologists (see Gould, 1977, pp. 1–7; Ritvo, p. 74).

It is no coincidence that Sterba, who began composing his dictionary in 1932, with Freud's approval, was writing during the same time span when Freud was writing *Moses and Monotheism* (1939a). Limitations of time and space prevent me from delving into the ideological, religious content of this monumental work, except as it impinges directly on the main subject matter of my inquiry; Numerous commentators (see Rice, Yerushalmi, among others) have written detailed critiques of *Moses and Monotheism* which examine Freud's construction of the historical Moses in relation to the history of religion and the author's life. My principal objective is to demonstrate how his conception of human evolution as it was formulated in 1915 is reflected in his thought processes near the end of his life, and how this conception, in turn, may be evaluated in today's psychoanalytic thinking and that of contemporary historians of science.

In section E of the third essay of *Moses and Monotheism* titled "Difficulties," Freud raises the question of how a religious tradition, such as that of Moses, can be transmitted from one generation to another in the absence of direct communication from one person to another. Central to his inquiry is an example given by the transmission between generations of a specific event, the purported murder of Moses at the hands of his followers, promulgated in a book by Ernst Sellin (1922). Freud states:

> "In order to make it easier for readers who do not desire or are not prepared to plunge into a complicated psychological state of affairs, I will anticipate the outcome of the investigation that is to follow. In my opinion there is an almost complete conformity in this respect between the individual and the group: In the group too an impression of the past is retained in unconscious memory-traces.
>
> (1939a, p. 94)

Having established an intimate connection between the psychology of the individual and that of the group, a topic that he had already discussed at length in *Group Psychology and the Analysis of the Ego* (1921c), he proceeds with his investigation:

> we become aware of the probability that what may be operative in the individual's psychical life may include not only what he has experienced himself but also things that were innately present in him at his birth, elements with a phylogenetic origin – an *archaic heritage.* … it consists in certain [innate] dispositions such as are characteristic of all living organisms … Since experience shows that there are distinctions… between individuals of the human species, the archaic heritage must include these distinctions; they represent what we recognize as the *constitutional* factor in the individual.
>
> (p. 98. Emphasis in original)

Pursuing this line of thought, Freud now brings the ontogenetic factor in the development of the psyche into play:

> When we study the reactions to early traumas, we are often quite surprised to find that they are not strictly limited to what the subject himself has really experienced but diverge from it in a way which fits in much better with the model of a phylogenetic event and, in general,

> can only be explained by such an influence. The behavior of neurotic children towards their parents in the Oedipus and castration complex abounds in such reactions, which seem justified in the individual case and only become intelligible phylogenetically – by their connection with the experience of earlier generations. … [The] evidential value [of this material] seems to me strong enough for me … to posit the assertion that the archaic heritage of human beings comprises not only dispositions but also subject matter – memory-traces of the experience of earlier generations.
>
> (p. 99)

As if anticipating an objection on the part of the reader to his postulating "an inherited tradition of this kind and not one transmitted by communication," he adds: "my position, no doubt, is made more difficult by the present attitude of biological science, which refuses to hear of the inheritance of acquired characters by succeeding generations" (p. 100). The reference here is to the now discredited theory of evolution formulated by Jean Baptiste de Lamarck ([1963] 1809) in the early nineteenth century.

Freud continues: "If we assume the survival of these memory traces in the archaic heritage, we have bridged the gulf between individual and group psychology: we can deal with peoples as we do with an individual neurotic" (p. 100). After conceding that "we have no stronger evidence for the presence of memory-traces in the archaic heritage than the residual phenomena of the work of analysis which call for a phylogenetic derivation" (p. 100), he comes to a succinct conclusion: "After this discussion I have no hesitation in declaring that men have always known… that they once possessed a primal father and killed him" (p. 101).

As an addendum to the foregoing argument, Freud poses "two further questions":

> First, under what conditions does a memory of this kind enter the archaic heritage? And, secondly, in what circumstances can it become active to consciousness… ? The answer to the first question is easy to formulate: the memory enters the archaic heritage if the event was important enough, or repeated often enough, or both. In the case of parricide both conditions are fulfilled. On the second question … A whole number of influences may be concerned…What is certainly of decisive importance, however, is the awakening of the forgotten memory-trace by a recent real repetition of the event. The murder of Moses was a repetition of this kind and, later, the supposed judicial murder of Christ.
>
> (p. 101)

In establishing a parallel between the psychology of the individual and that of the group, with its roots in the "archaic heritage" Freud put himself in a position to describe historical processes in terms of a "real repetition" of a past event, which occurs as a combination of traumatic events in the history of the individual and the group and the repetition of those experiences in each over the course of time. In so doing he made use of both recapitulation theory and the inheritance of acquired characteristics as adumbrated in his "phylogenetic fantasy" of 1915. In the case of Moses the principal traumatic event was his murder at the hands of his followers, which was subjected to the forces of repression for several generations, only to reemerge in a distorted form, condensed with experiences of the groups that followed, who would coalesce into the cultural and historical nucleus of the Jewish people. Freud describes this process succinctly under the heading of "The Historical Premiss":

> Modern historical research has been able to extract two facts from the obscurity which the biblical narrative has left, or rather created, at this point. The first of these facts, discovered by Ernst Sellin, is that the Jews, who ... were headstrong and unruly towards their law-giver and leader, rose against him one day, killed him and threw off the religion of the Aten which had been imposed on them, just as the Egyptians had thrown it off earlier. The second fact, demonstrated by Eduard Meyer [1906], is that those Jews who had returned from Egypt united later on with closely related tribes in the region between Palestine, the Sinai Peninsula and Arabia, and there, in a well-watered locality named Kadesh, they took on a new religion, the worship of the volcano God Yahweh. Soon after this they were ready to invade Canaan as conquerors.
>
> (pp. 60f.)

Having established that the union of the two groups at Kadesh and the subsequent merging of two disparate belief systems (the Yahwistic and the Mosaic)--which both share an allegiance to a single god--into a single tradition, with the latter eclipsing the former, Freud attempts to account for this monumental transformation in both psychological and historical terms:

> Pious believers... say that the idea of a single god produced such an overwhelming effect on men because it is a portion of the eternal *truth* which, long concealed, came to light at last and was then bound to carry everyone along with it... We too would like to accept this solution. But we are brought up by a doubt. ...We too believe that the pious solution contains the truth – but the *historical* truth and not the *material* truth. ...We had assumed that the religion of Moses was to begin with rejected and half-forgotten and afterwards broke through as a tradition. We are now assuming that this process was being repeated then

> for a second time. When Moses brought the people the idea of a single god, it was not a novelty but signified the revival of an experience in the primaeval ages of the human family which had long vanished from men's conscious memory. But it had been so important and had produced or paved the way for such deeply penetrating changes in men's life that we cannot avoid believing that it had left behind it in the human mind some permanent traces, which can be compared to a tradition.
>
> (p. 129)

Freud's conception of a historical tradition, be it religious or otherwise, is made up of two elements: 1) actual events, either isolated or in series, which have been communicated over time orally by some individuals and recorded by others; and 2) innate qualities residing in the individual psyche that transmit the memory of the events in question through generations and subject them to distortion, amplification and/or concealment. In the case of Moses the events in question involve the material truth concerning his origins, his character, the course of his life, and his relations with his followers, and the historical truth as presented by the generations that created the tradition that was formed in his name. Both elements have been and are still a subject of controversy.

In his critique of Freud's twelfth metapsychology paper, Yerushalmi writes:

> In this extraordinary document... Freud attempted nothing less than a historical view of the neuroses as phylogenetically inherited mechanisms originally developed by all of humanity in order to meet the real, perilous exigencies of the Ice Age and its aftermath. ... Nowhere is Freud's Lamarckism more striking and radical than in *Moses and Monotheism*... it is one thing to imagine the formation of a phylogenetic heritage in the remotest prehistoric ages when, ostensibly the structures of the human psyche were still in an early and fluid process of evolution, and certain overwhelming and universal experiences, repeated again and again over enormous periods of time, eventually left biological imprints that could somehow be transmitted somatically to future generations.
>
> Here, however, trauma in the form of a unique cluster of historical events, their encoding within the genetic legacy of a particular group, collective repression, and the 'return of the repressed' all take place in relatively recent historical time within a brief span of some five to eight centuries. Moreover, not only the traumatic slaying of Moses, but the content of his religious teaching is alleged to have undergone this fateful and intricate process
>
> (pp. 30f.)

Citing Freud's continued reliance on recapitulation and psycho-Lamarckism as the two "linchpins" of his historical constructions, Gould, in a recently written critique of the unpublished draft "Overview of the Transference Neuroses," (1987b) writes:

> Freud's theory requires the passage to heredity of events that occurred tens of thousands of years ago at most. But such events – anxiety at approaching ice sheets, castration of sons, and murder of fathers – have no hereditary impact. However traumatic, they do not affect the eggs and sperm of parents and therefore cannot pass into heredity under Mendelian and Darwinian rules. Even if they could, the time available is far too short, for Darwinism is a slow process of accumulating small variants generation by generation.
>
> (p. 18)

Extending his critique to include what he considers to be the views of contemporary psychoanalysts, he continues:

> Since most commentators have not grasped the logic of Freud's theory for failure to recognize the roles of Lamarckism and recapitulation, they are left in something of a dilemma, particularly if they are generally sympathetic to Freud. Without these linchpins, the theory sounds plain crazy. Could Freud really mean that these events of recent history somehow got into the inheritance of children [we might add: "and groups"] and the fixated behavior of neurotics? Consequently, a muted or kindly tradition has arisen among commentators for viewing Freud's claims as merely symbolic. He didn't really mean that exiled sons actually killed their father and that Oedipal complexes truly reenact a specific event of our past. Freud's words, they claim, are just colorful imagery that provides insight into the psychological meaning of neurosis.
>
> (p. 18)

In his adamant rejection of this "kindly" tradition, Gould concludes: "Freud's writing gives no indication that he considered his phylogenetic speculation as anything but a potentially true account of what actually happened. If he had only meant these ideas as metaphor, why work out such a consistency with biological theory based on Lamarckism and recapitulation?" (p. 18).

In his monumental biography of Freud, Jones (1957) prefigures Gould's critique when he writes:

> Freud never gave up a jot of his belief in the inheritance of acquired characters. How immovable he was in the matter I discovered during a talk I had with him in the last year of his life over a sentence I wished

> him to alter in the Moses book in which he expressed the Lamarckian view in universal terms. I told him he had of course the right to hold any opinion he liked in his own field of psychology… but begged him to omit the passage where he applied it to the whole field of biological evolution, since no responsible biologist regarded it as tenable any longer.
>
> (p. 313)

We know that Freud refused to comply with Jones' request, if only because to alter a single passage in *Moses and Monotheism* would presumably have necessitated his abandoning the Lamarckian concept altogether, which would have been difficult, given its prominence in several of his seminal works written earlier, from *Totem and Taboo* on; but at the conclusion of his account of the creation of "the Moses book," Jones softens the impact of his earlier condemnation with the following qualifying remark:

> Although we have found occasion to criticize Freud's Lamarckian assumptions on the transmission of the effects of experiences this by no means disposes of his theory of an inherited sense of guilt or the importance of transmission by tradition. There are alternative presentations possible that would preserve the essence of his conclusions.
>
> (p. 374)

One such alternative presentation might be represented by Assmann's response to Yerushalmi's critique of Freud's psycho-Lamarckism cited above, which, he concedes,

> is correct, of course, but Freud's question is not, in the first place, how these memories could have been transmitted, but how the memory of Moses and his monotheism could have met with such enormous resonance eight hundred years after the hypothetical lifetime of Moses.
>
> It is a theory of trauma or, in the terminology of Aleida Assmann, of 'impact and resonance.' Some incomprehensively overwhelming 'impact event' creates a kind of resonance in such a form that later events are experienced as a return of the original event. This, however, is not a matter of centuries but of generations.
>
> (p. 66)

Assmann applies the concept of "impact and resonance" to the experience of the Egyptians in the wake of Akhenaten's imposition of the Aten religion on them:

> The most important evidence for the traumatic character of the Amarna experience… is to be found in Egyptian sources only about a thousand

> years later. In this case, we are fully justified in speaking of repression, latency, and the return of the repressed. … The notion of 'resonance' refers to the human inclination to comprehend new experiences in the light of past experiences serving as model or schema. In this way, traditional Judaism used to term historical catastrophes*hurbân*, a term that originally designated the destruction of the Second Temple. The term 'impact,' by contrast, refers to events that exceed all traditional models and schemata and produce speechlessness. Such an event was the one that later came to be called *shoah*, or 'holocaust.' Maybe the Amarna experience was the same kind of impact event for the Egyptians, becoming accessible to verbal articulation only much later. This happened, in fact, six hundred years later in a historical situation that had many things in common with the historical context in which the Exodus narrative emerged. Some vague memory traces of Amarna must have survived in Egyptian oral tradition What reactivated these traces was the experience of four devastating invasions in the first half of the seventh century that not only destroyed the Egyptian temples and hijacked the cult images, but also forced it into vassaldom.
>
> (p. 70)

Although Assmann presents a persuasive case in demonstrating that the memory of traumatic events in the history of a people can be reactivated in later generations of the same people, his invoking of the oral tradition as the principal mechanism of this transmission and a similarity between the respective events in question lends little support for Freud's conception of phylogenetic memory and its effects on individuals and groups. Notwithstanding the similarity, the historical connection between the trauma of the Amarna experience and that of the Assyrian invasions bears no direct relation to the guilt-laden trauma generated by the purported murder of Moses at the hands of his followers and its recapitulation in the religious traditions of the Jewish people.

Nonetheless, it would be an error on the part of both historians and psychologists to disregard completely the role of biological evolution on the motivation of individuals and groups in the course of history. In her content-rich discussion of the historico-scientific dimension of the "Overview of the Transference Neuroses," Grubrich-Simitis observes:

> The traumatic real experience in Freud's early conception of the etiology of hysteria appears in fully developed psychoanalytic theory set back into the distant past of the prehistory of the species, that is, transposed from the ontogenetic to the phylogenetic dimension. When viewed from this perspective, the psycho-Lamarckian components of metapsychology are something like a bracket between two stages in the development of Freudian theory. For him to give them up would presumably also have meant to play down psychoanalysis, at least to

> question its claim to universal validity as a fundamental transcultural statement on the human condition. Furthermore, the postulate helped Freud bridge "the gulf between individual and group psychology."
>
> (p. 99)

In commenting on the history of the concept of evolution itself, particularly as it existed when Freud was in the process of putting his "phylogenetic fantasy" into written form, she states:

> [We] must realize that the explanatory concepts of Darwin and Lamarck were not originally considered antagonistic models. While Darwinism was in its ascendancy, the investigations of Jean-Baptiste Lamarck were rediscovered as a significant pioneering achievement on the way to a scientific theory of evolution...
>
> (pp. 100f.)

In the first paragraph of the first chapter of his book, *Time's Arrow, Time's Cycle*, Gould credits Freud with having "shattered yet another facet of an original hope for our own transcendent importance in the universe. ... the solace that, though evolved from a lowly ape, we at least possessed rational minds..." but that in so doing, "[he] neglected the great temporal limitation imposed by geology upon human importance – the discovery of 'deep time'... What could be more comforting... than the traditional concept of a young earth, ruled by human will within days of its origin. How threatening, by contrast, the notion of an almost incomprehensible immensity, with human habitation restricted to a millimicrosecond at the very end!" (1987, pp. 1f.).

Although Freud clearly did not believe that the earth was ruled by human will within days of its origin, Gould does lay bare a fundamental flaw in Freud's notion that the hereditary component of the dispositions to modern neuroses could have been formed within the relatively short time span of the Ice Ages, which is measured in thousands of years, in contrast to the entire course of biological evolution, which is measured in millions of years. Modern evolutionary biologists are in general agreement that evolution takes place at the cellular level, with minute changes that can take place over long periods of time, eventually producing major variations in individuals of a species which are in turn either perpetuated in their progeny or eliminated in the process of natural selection. By the same token, it is inconceivable that the memory of a single event, like the murder of Moses, along with the reaction-formations that accompanied the act, could have been lodged in the germ-plasm of his followers and emerged generations later in the religious practices of their descendants.

At the same time, we would be remiss in dismissing altogether the role of hereditary factors in forming the motivations of individuals and groups and their effects on the course of history. What Freud, Darwin,

Lamarck and most modern biologists and historians all have in common is their acknowledgment of the fact that all human beings are animals, descended from primitive life forms that existed in the remotest past ages, endowed with specific traits that allowed them to adapt to the exigencies of the struggle for survival. In this respect, we, as human beings, are no exception. When one speaks of specific aspects of the human condition, then, does it really matter how these traits were acquired or when they originated? Given the tentative nature of Freud's theorizing in general and the fluidity of his thinking about the origins of religion in particular, is it not sufficient to acknowledge that the instinct to kill is lodged in the genetic makeup of all humans, as it is in all higher animals, and that it is immaterial whether the followers of Moses actually murdered him or merely entertained the wish to do so? There is ample evidence, both in the Biblical narrative and the historical record of all cultures, of instances where individuals or groups of individuals either attempted to murder their superiors and/or succeeded in doing so. No further support is necessary to lend credence to Freud's declaration that "men have always known … that they once possessed a primal father and killed him" (1939a, p. 101).

Frank Sulloway, historian of science and colleague of Stephen Jay Gould's at Harvard, comments, using Kuhn's (1962) oft-cited terminology:

> [H]istory is inevitably harsh in its assessment of those individuals who have sought to transform "preparadigmatic" into 'paradigmatic' sciences. Such was the nature of Freud's endeavor. If he was only partially successful, one must still acknowledge that his synthetic approach and his theoretical daring were highly appropriate to the particular historical context in which he expressed them. Perhaps only Aristotle and Darwin have equaled Freud's marriage of theory and observation in the broad realm of the life sciences.
>
> (1992, p. 500)

In commenting on the subtitle of his seminal biography of Luther, Erikson (1962) writes:

> This "Study in Psychoanalysis and History" will reevaluate a segment of history (here the youth of a great reformer) by using psychoanalysis as a historical tool; but it will also, here and there, throw light on psychoanalysis as a tool of history. … As a method of observation it takes history; as a system of ideas it makes history.
>
> (pp. 16f.)

If we compare Erikson's endeavor in constructing the life of Luther with that of Freud's in constructing the life of Moses we note a number of similarities, the most noteworthy of which is that of methodology, as referenced in Erikson's subtitle and the original German title of Freud's work, *Der Mann Moses und die Monotheistische Religion*, which, translated literally, means "The Man Moses and Monotheistic Religion." In both instances, the biographer uses the methodology of psychoanalysis as a tool in illuminating the at times conflicted motivation of a single individual in relation to an external reality, the consequences of which helped determine the course of history. The most notable difference in the two instances is that Erikson had considerable documentary evidence on which to base his constructions, much of which stemmed directly from his subject's own spoken and written words, whereas Freud had to rely on secondary written sources that were chronologically and spatially remote from the events that they described and otherwise unreliable largely on account of tendentious, wishful motives on the part of their authors. Consequently, Freud had to rely more on psychoanalytic theory, derived from clinical experience, and less on extant historical evidence by which to support his conclusions.

The last paragraph of his paper on technique, "Constructions in Analysis" (1937d), published two years before the publication of *Moses and Monotheism*, resonates with Freud's construction of the origins of monotheism and that of the image of the man who helped make it accessible to large portions of the Western world:

> If we consider mankind as a whole and substitute it for the single human individual, we discover that it too has developed delusions which are inaccessible to logical criticism and which contradict reality. If, in spite of this, they are able to exert an extraordinary power over men, investigation leads us to the same explanation as in the case of the single individual. They owe their power to the element of *historical truth* which they have brought up from the repression of the forgotten and primaeval past.
>
> (p. 269; emphasis in original)

The nature of that primeval past and the role that it plays in determining the elusive truth of the human condition have been and will remain a subject of ongoing inquiry.

By way of an epilogue to the preceding, I would like to offer the following excerpts from Martin Luther King Jr.'s last sermon, delivered in Memphis, Tennessee, on April 3, 1968:

> If I were standing at the beginning of time, with the possibility of general and panoramic view of the whole human history up to now, and the Almighty said to me, 'Martin Luther King, which age would you like to live in?' – I would take my mental flight through, or rather across the Red Sea, through the wilderness on toward the Promised Land and in spite of its magnificence, I wouldn't stop there. …

> And then I got to Memphis. … Well, I don't know what will happen now. … But it doesn't matter to me now, Because I've been to the mountaintop and I don't mind. … And He's allowed me to go up to the mountain. And I've looked over. And I've seen the Promised Land. I may not get there with you, but I want you to know tonight that we, as a people, will get to the Promised Land.

Martin Luther King was murdered on April 4, 1968 by James Earl Ray, an avowed racist and convicted felon. Ray's motives and the events and circumstances surrounding his act have been widely publicized and commented on, and continue to be the subject of controversy. What has been less widely publicized is the fact that King narrowly escaped death in an earlier attempt on his life at the hands of Izola Curry, who stabbed him with a steel letter opener at a book signing in Harlem on September 20, 1958. She was tried for attempted murder, diagnosed as a paranoid schizophrenic, and committed to the New York State Hospital for the Criminally Insane.

King never knew his assailants personally, nor did either of them know the other. Yet there is a commonality in the respective experiences of each of the principals which leads one to want to reveal the material truth contained in them.

References

Assmann, J. (2014). *From Akhenaten to Moses. Ancient Egypt and Religious Change.* New York: American University in Cairo Press. Cairo, Egypt.

Erikson, E. (1962). *Young Man Luther. A Study in Psychoanalysis and History.* New York: Norton.

Falzeder, E. & Brabant, E. Eds. (1996). *The Correspondence of Sigmund Freud and Sándor Ferenczi, Volume II, 1914–1919.* (P.Hoffer, Trans., A Hoffer, Intro.). Cambridge: Harvard University Press.

Freud, S. (1912–1913). *Totem and Taboo. S. E.* 13: 1–161. London: Hogarth.

Freud, S. (1915c). Instincts and their vicissitudes. *S. E.* 14: 117–140. London: Hogarth.

Freud, S. (1915d). Repression. *S. E.* 14: 141–158. London: Hogarth.

Freud, S. (1915e). The unconscious. *S. E.* 14: 159–216. London: Hogarth.

Freud, S. (1917d). A metapsychological supplement to the theory of dreams. *S. E.* 14: 222–235. London: Hogarth.

Freud, S. (1917e). Mourning and melancholia. *S. E.* 14: 237–260. London: Hogarth.

Freud, S. (1921c). *Group Psychology and the Analysis of the Ego. S. E.*, 18: 65–143. London: Hogarth.

Freud, S. (1937d). Constructions in analysis. *S. E.* 23: 256–269. London: Hogarth.

Freud, S. (1939a). *Moses and Monotheism. S. E.* 23: 7–137. London: Hogarth.

Freud, S. (1987 [1915]). *A Phylogenetic Fantasy: Overview of the Transference Neuroses*, I. Grubrich-Simitis (Ed.), A. & P. Hoffer (Trans.). Cambridge: Harvard University Press.

Gould, S. (1977). *Ontogeny and Phylogeny.* Cambridge: Harvard University Press.

Gould, S. (1987a). *Time's Arrow, Time's Cycle.* Cambridge: Harvard University Press.
Gould, S. (1987b). Freud's phylogenetic fantasy. Only great thinkers are allowed to fail greatly. *Natural Hist ory, 12*: 10–16.
Grubrich-Simitis, I. (1987). Metapsychology and metabiology. In: Freud (1987 [1915]), pp. 75–107.
Haeckel, E. (1868). *Natürliche Schöpfungsgeschichte.* Berlin: Georg Reimer.
Jones, E. (1957). *The Life and Work of Sigmund Freud,* Vol. 3. New York: Basic Books.
Kuhn, T. (1962). *The Structure of Scientific Revolutions.* Chicago: University of ChicagoPress.
Lamarck, J. B. (1963 [1809]). *Zoological Philosophy: An Exposition with Regard to the Natural History of Animals.* New York: Hafner.
Meyer, E. (1906). *Die Israeliten und ihre Nachbarstämme.* Halle: M. Niemeyer.
Rice, E. (1990). *Freud and Moses. The Long Journey Home.* Albany: State University of NewYork Press.
Ritvo, L. (1990). *Darwin's Influence on Freud. A Tale of Two Sciences.* New Haven: Yale University Press.
Sellin, E. (1922). *Mose und seine Bedeutung für die israelitisch-jüdische Religionsgeschichte.* Leipzig: A. Deichertsche Verlagsbuchhandlung.
Sterba, R. (2013). *The First Dictionary of Psychoanalysis. A Gift for Sigmund Freud's 80th Birthday.* P. Hoffer (Trans.) The International Psychoanalysis Library. London: Karnac.
Sulloway, F. (1992). *Freud, Biologist of the Mind. Beyond the Psychoanalytic Legend.* Cambridge: Harvard University Press.
Yerushalmi, Y. (1991). *Freud's Moses. Judaism Terminable and Interminable.* New Haven: Yale University Press.

Editor's Introduction to Chapter 3

Lawrence J. Brown

Noting that Freud's last book, *Moses and Monotheism*, was written during the upsurge of Nazism in Germany and Austria during the 1930s, Laurence Kahn aptly begins her chapter stating that "*Moses and Monotheism* is a book of despair… infinitely deeper than that which followed Titus' destruction of the temple." We may wonder what could be more profoundly disturbing then the razing of this second temple, rebuilt in 350 BC to replace the first temple built in Jerusalem in 957 BC that was destroyed by the Babylonians? Kahn's reply, I believe, is that Nazism and the destruction of European culture, and Jewish culture in particular, in the Second World War is a despair that exceeds in depth and breadth all previous acts of cruelty to the Jewish people. Freud, too, was appalled by the seemingly boundless viciousness of the Nazis and could have easily linked this to his theory of the death instinct, but Khan notes that he chose instead to observe and describe what he witnessed. He soon came to understand what Kahn's title to this essay tells us: that anything is "Probable in Nazi Times."

Kahn also reminds us of Freud's earlier writings about the nature of *Civilization and Its Discontents* and that what we call culture is constantly in tension with our biology, "In the end, it is the biological that regulates our dealings with civilization… [and] man's evolution is animal, subject only to the laws of adaptation and its accidents" (this volume). She also reminds the reader of Freud's observations that group processes under certain circumstances resemble psychotic phenomena in the individual patient. Freud, too, despaired that culture and society could so easily be uprooted and Kahn deftly quotes his haunting observation that this time was a "specially remarkable period…[in which] we find to our astonishment that progress has allied itself with barbarism" (Freud, 1939).

In summary, Laurence Kahn offers us an insightful and unsettling overview of a world gone crazy – the Probable in Nazi Times – in which hatred was unleashed and the Law, whether that of Moses' Tables of the Law or secular law, was perverted and 'purified' in accord with Nazi principles of German superiority. The reader will surely be moved by this chapter and likely see parallels to current cultural developments.

DOI: 10.4324/9781003272045-6

3 The Probable in Nazi Times

The Opposing Fates of the Mystical and the Law*

Laurence Kahn

Political Desolation

The Man Moses and Monotheistic Religion[1] is a book of despair. When books are burned and they are making ready to burn people, what remains of writing and the law? When Freud apologizes to his readers in the brief preface to the Hebrew translation of the *Introductory Lectures on Psychoanalysis*, he already knows that this despair is infinitely deeper than that which followed the destruction of the Temple by Titus. Did Moses and the Prophets understand these lessons?[2] From this point of view, the final leg of Freud's journey, which stretches from 1934 to 1939, seems to be a direct development of the 1932 epistolary exchange between Freud and Einstein on the disaster of law[3] and the eruption of war. It is likewise wholly in keeping with the thirty-fifth of the *New Lectures*, on the "Weltanschauung." In more than one way, *The Man Moses* is a political text.

Lethal violence repeated, at the time engulfing the entire social sphere, does more than engender disillusion. It does more than constrain renouncing the ultimate vague hopes of rationality which guided the man of the Enlightenment. Between the inquiry on the "creation of a people" by a "man"[4] and the examination of the psychic roots of religious belief, Freud quietly questions the sources of the devastating explosiveness blowing across the Germanic countries. Especially as in this instance he does not make any shortcuts: at no time does he make use of the concept of the death drive to account for the abuse suffered by the Jews and the destructiveness troubling his compatriots.

Perhaps this is why *The Man Moses* is doubly a book of despair. The return of the trauma and the development of the theory of the *après-coup* regarding groups and culture in effect attacks from the rear the sort of promise inherent to murder. Up till then, from the initial use of the Oedipus the King tragedy through *Civilization and Its Discontents*, murder and the threat of its repetition inserted guilt into the very bedrock of the human community. Whatever the reworking of the model of the psychic apparatus, they would guarantee the psychic conditions of possible repression, the subterranean stay of the social and civilizational pact.

DOI: 10.4324/9781003272045-7

To be sure, this pillar is extremely precarious. When in *Civilization and Its Discontents* Freud asserts that we are pacifists by necessity, that culture is but a material expression of the animal's survival instinct, a poor defense against our compulsion to exterminate to the last,[5] and that concerning enthusiasm there remains but the duty to reject it,[6] he tears culture away from the sphere of the life of the mind. It is, as all human creation, taken up in the snares of the constraints of natural law. Biology ultimately regulates our tangles with civilization, which prohibits us from carrying out our extinction "without further diversions."[7]

Freud then broke not only with Hegel but, whatever one might say, with Lamarck. To Lamarck – who postulated the existence of an internal orthogenetic force, a law of progressive development tending toward perfection[8] – Freud in essence replied that man's evolution is animal, subject only to the laws of adaption and its accidents, despite all the illusions that he erects in order to protest against his subjection to nature. And to Hegel, he denies the illusion of progress supported by the infinite power of Reason.[9] Against the dialectical reversals of negativity which characterize this process as development, against the revolutionary negation of the account which makes murder out to be the moment of the achievement of freedom,[10] and against this truth which would reside and disclose itself in the temporal process itself, Freud rebels in opposing a scientific explanation of development. Scientific, because this explanation concedes nothing to the illusions of a scarcely secularized religion which, purporting to be based on history, speaks to us in truth about a higher purpose having as its end the self-realization of the spirit. Against this belief, he held that development arises only out of the struggle which the repeated search for primary satisfaction and the resistances erecting barriers to repress it engage in unceasingly.

Freud was very clear in *Civilization and Its Discontents*. The root cause of the confrontation is not found in the opposition of the originary drives, Eros and death. It concerns "a dispute within the economics of the libido, comparable to the contest concerning the distribution of libido between ego and objects."[11] Whereas it is as a direct consequence of the evocation of this founding conflict that Freud envisages the "analogy between the process of civilization and the path of individual development," adding that the "superego of an epoch of civilization has an origin similar to that of an individual."[12] In both cases, the desire for murder and its interdiction determine the establishment of moral consciousness and the law without which men cannot live in society.

But this does not necessarily mean that the legislation is shielded from the danger of being itself but an illusion.

> Besides, have you learned nothing from history? [...] Surely you remember the French Revolution and Robespierre? And you must also remember how short-lived and miserably ineffectual the experiment

> was? The same experiment is being repeated in Russia at the present time, and we need not feel curious as to its outcome.[13]

At the center of this debate, we recall the skirmish between Freud and his imaginary interlocutor in *The Future of an Illusion*, which does not miss drawing out the paradox inherent to psychoanalysis' discourse of truth: "you," Freud has him say, "emerge as an enthusiast [the *Schwärmer*] who allows himself to be carried away by illusions, and I stand for the claims of reason, the rights of skepticism."[14] In other words, what are progressive prejudices and their will to universalism worth? How can the voice of reason make itself heard? So it is that at the end of "Why War?" Freud calls for the "dictatorship of reason,"[15] the only one capable of countering religious belief as it forges a more solid unifying authority and tie. We gauge the tension here in which Freud is caught between a "dictatorship" best able to gather together ungovernable humans and a drive program capable of protecting the species from its self-destruction.

In truth, each time that Freud returns to culture in terms of a program through putting the survival of the species at the heart of cultural aspiration, we observe him relying on a teleological perspective which simultaneously orders the fate of each individual. In his view, the task of education is but a *Nachhilfe*, assistance *après-coup*, and educators are but the executants of the program in charge of the repression necessary for the edification of moral forces.[16] But the construction of these levees against drive violence fundamentally belongs to a process internal to humanity. Which Freud says explicitly when he maintains the existence of spontaneous repression among children. Human spontaneity is then related to "a primæval and prehistoric demand" which "has at last become part of the organized and inherited endowment of mankind."[17]

However, as always when it is a matter of relating individual to collective aspirations, Freud is overcome by doubt: "The use of teleology as a heuristic hypothesis has its dubious side," he writes. In "any instance one can never tell whether one has hit upon a 'harmony' or a 'disharmony.' It is the same as when one drives a nail into the wall of a room: one cannot be certain whether one is going to come up against lath and plaster or brick-work."[18]

Science or Probable?

Is this the reason why the question of science and truth is asked in such a sharp manner in *The Man Moses*? "Not even the most tempting probability is a protection against error; even if all the parts of a problem seem to fit together like the pieces of a jig-saw puzzle, one must reflect that what is probable is not necessarily the truth and that the truth is not always probable. And lastly, it did not seem attractive to find oneself classed with the schoolmen and Talmudists who delight in exhibiting their ingenuity without regard to how remote from reality their thesis may be."[19]

Beginning with the first manuscript version, dated August 9, 1934 and rediscovered by Yerushalmi in the Freud Archives in the Library of Congress in Washington, the probable is present, and it is accompanied by this caveat. The question of knowing what kind of truth his method attains already torments Freud. Even if the indifference to the reality of the Talmudists is lacking, the shadow of the scientific critique nonetheless looms: "I have been trained to the careful scrutiny of a certain domain of phenomena. To me fiction and invention are easily associated with the blemish of error."[20] Consequently, the truth value of this "historical novel" is impossible to determine since "factual evidence can only in small measure be replaced by deductions and speculations."[21]

And indeed it is remarkable that the noun, *vraisemblance* (*Wahrscheinlichkeit*), as well as the adjective, *vraisemblable* (*wahrscheinlich*), is given prominence from beginning to end. This does not appear in the English translation, which renders these terms by "probability" and "probable," terms which overlook the root *wahr**/*vrai** present in German and French – or *true** in English. This is why the hypothesis of Moses's being Egyptian is "probable" (*GW* 16, p. 113). As is "probable" the reverence of a single sun god by Akhenaton in the hymns attributed to him (pp. 121–122). As is "probable" the fanatical desire for vengeance of the clerics oppressed by Amon. Yet again "probable" is the hypothesis that between Moses's death and the founding of the religion in Kadesh two generations had gone by (p. 139). It is not very "probable" on the other hand that Moses could take part in the events in Kadesheven if his life was not shortened (p. 149). The stretch of time between the appearance of a new teaching and its acceptance by the community however is "probable": witness Darwinian theory (p. 170). Lastly, is "probable" the hypothesis of two stages and the resurgence of monotheism, if judged by the preservation in the Homeric poems of a largely prior cultural flowering dating from the Minoan-Mycenaean period (pp. 174–175). In short, is "probable" the fact that what is active in the individual's psychic life does not fall under content experienced alone by the individual himself but also from elements originating in an archaic, indeed, a phylogenetic heritage (p. 204). This is why the probable gradually proves to be the buttress of the analogy.

But the question of the probable touches on something more serious. It bears on what may be the role of a "man," even if he were great, and his power to create a people. A crucial question which engages the status of the Jewish people at a time when the Germanic countries, dominated by anti-Semitic frenzy, are themselves transfixed by a "man," a *Führer*.[22] What determines the longevity of the Jewish people, the resistance to time of its specific characteristics? What jurisdiction does its conception of election fall within, including, at its greatest expense? If the debate on what it means to be a Jew when you are a godless Jew underlies the whole of *The Man Moses* – let's not forget that Freud appeared to decide not to have his sons circumcised[23] – Freud conjointly questions the historical conditions in which a people establish, under the aegis of monotheism, this relationship specific to the law (*loi*) which was the commandments. He questions this founding at the very moment when murder organized and made legitimate collectively modifies the base of the interdiction radically. As Hannah Arendt will put it,

> [...] Hitler-Germany demonstrated that an ideology which almost consciously reversed the command "Thou shalt not kill" need meet no overwhelming resistance from a conscience trained in the Western tradition. On the contrary, Nazi ideology often was able to reverse the functioning of this conscience [...].[24]

This is what Freud is witness to: this "remarkable times" in which we "find to our astonishment that progress has allied itself with barbarism."[25] A horrifying astonishment which, at the very end of his work, requires the intelligence and courage to note the irremediable uncoupling of scientific progress and progress in the life of the mind. It is quite precisely with regard to this dreadful observation that Freud reshapes his understanding of group pathology on psychosis, religious phenomena included –even modifying thereby the former understanding of belief as produced by neurosis alone. Adorno, Waelder, and Fenichel will seize on this hypothesis at the symposium on anti-Semitism organized in San Francisco by Horkheimer and Simmel in 1949. What in reality is at stake is a turn in the perception of the civilizing process, the psychotic rent of belief weighing far greater than religious conviction.

Delirium and Truth

It is with the writing of *The Man Moses* – and Freud notes as such clearly in the 1935 postscript to his *Autobiographical Study* – that the perspective is modified:

> In *The Future of an Illusion* I expressed an essentially negative valuation of religion. Later, I found a formula which did better justice to it; while granting that its power lies in the truth which contains, I showed that truth was not a material but a historical truth.[26]

Now it is precisely this formulation which compromises *The Man Moses* since one may simply consider the hypothesis making Moses an Egyptian as "a product of the imagination [*Phantasie*] and too remote from reality."[27] Whence the necessity of a solid historical foothold making it possible to rule out suspicion. And in fact, beginning with the initial moment when

Jones tried to convince Freud to abandon his Lamarckism – in the name of a possible accusation of guilt by association between Lamarckism and Bolshevism which ran the risk of doing harm to psychoanalysis – numerous and virulent were the criticisms addressed by historians. I'm thinking notably of Yerushalmi's in the final chapter of *Zakhor*, "Modern Dilemmas: Historiography and Its Discontents."

One may tell oneself in order to quell the discord that Freud does not wholly invent the existence of the two Moses, that he is going back to Schiller's text, "Moses's Mission," that he takes it over via the hypotheses of Reinhold (for whom Moses is ethnically a Hebrew but culturally an Egyptian), that last but not least he is referring to Goethe's essay, "Israel in the Desert" – which attempts to separate poetry and truth from what comes down to us out of the Old Testament tradition. But there is no getting around it. The misunderstanding is complete, since Freudian "historical truth" has absolutely nothing to do with the historical method but everything with the repetition compulsion, and that the "probable," opening up the collective field to the action of the unconscious, gains purchase on the hypothesis of memory traces which Freud infers based on the assessment of a return of the repressed: murder.

Thus the criticism does not originate in the frail nature of "material truth" on which Freud bases himself, resting on a modicum of tangible proofs. The historians, Marc Bloch, as it happens, know this very well: "Historical facts are inherently psychological facts,"[28] just as they know that in history there are no "facts endowed, if by any extraordinary chance, with an in fact flat-out defined, simple, irreducible existence."[29] No, the difficulty floated by this book, about which Freud says by turns that it is a novel and that it is not one, lies elsewhere. It is due to the status accorded to psychic reality in history, which further comfortably goes past the bounds of a history of mentalities: can an essay on the hallucinatory actualization in the long term of history avoid the suspicion of being itself a hallucinatory actualization?

Freud is conscious of the problem's amplitude. At this very time, in "Constructions in Analysis," he elaborates on the idea that madness not only proceeds methodically but that it likewise contains an element of *historical truth*. Now similarly this individual historical truth is not based on a historical conception of the memorial temporality of events. On the contrary, it is nourished by the infantile source of what has been taken from conscious history such as those memories in the form of hallucinations – including among patients in no way psychotic – which appear as the return of a forgotten event from one's very earliest years. Delirium, adds Freud, must therefore not be countered by attempting to convince the ill person of the contradiction that opposes him to reality but quite rather by lending its full worth to the unconscious truth contained in the delusional hallucination and its distortions. Still more: "The delusions of patients appear to me to be the equivalents of the constructions which we build up in the course of an analytic treatment – attempts at explanation and cure, though it is true that these, under the conditions of a psychosis, can do no more than replace the fragment of reality that is being disavowed in the present by another fragment that had already been disavowed in the past."[30] They are equivalents since, in both cases, the construction restores a lost fragment of lived history, that which the delirium substitutes for rejected reality. Yet this operation is specifically the one Freud carries out in *The Man Moses* – which he emphasizes in "Constructions in Analysis" when he ponders the idea that historical truth, like a phantom, similarly inhabits the delirious beliefs of the masses, whether religious or not: "If we consider mankind as a whole and substitute it for the single individual, we discover that it too has developed delusions which are inaccessible to logical criticism and which contradict reality. If, in spite of this, they are able to exert an extraordinary power over men, investigation leads us to the same explanation as in the case of the single individual. They owe their power to the element of *historical truth* which they have brought up from the repression of the forgotten and primæval past."[31]

At this point the association between delirium and truth is at its apogee, and Freud contemplates this head-on in *The Man Moses*:

> It is worth specially stressing the fact that each portion which returns from oblivion asserts itself with peculiar force, exercises an incomparably powerful influence on people in the mass, and raises an irresistible claim to truth against which logical objections remain powerless: a kind of "*credo quia absurdum*." This remarkable feature can only be understood on the pattern of the delusions of psychotics.

With the exception that religious beliefs, as a phenomenon of the masses, "escape the curse of isolation."[32]

"At which point even the most ardent and loyal admirer of Freud can only whisper to himself, '*Certum, quia absurdum est*,'"[33] summarizes Yerushalmi, who finds it difficult to imagine that Freud is referring not only to religious dogma but is more broadly considering the attempts "to master the sensory world [...] by means of the wishful world."[34] Might Hitler's masses likewise not "escape the curse of isolation"? When in the 35th introductory lecture Freud emphasizes that ethical demands which religion stresses "are indispensable to human society" but that "it is dangerous to link obedience to them with religious faith," what infantile "consolations" is he referring to?[35] How is he able to consider the relationship between the disintegration of the law (*loi*) and the delirious conviction taking possession of the German masses?

This question rises to the surface when, concerning the figure of the "great man," Freud underscores that group phenomenon take shape in the encounter with the kind of figure capable of satisfying "a powerful need for an authority who can be admired, before whom one bows down, by whom one is ruled and perhaps even ill-treated."[36] To be sure Freud is talking to us about Moses. But the underside of this figure is the one who dominates the psychic and material life of Freud's contemporaries, Hitler. Wouldn't the veneration of the *Führer* by a people passionately merged into a singular being call for the elucidation of the transition between individual and collective pathology? The nostalgia for the father who inhabits each individual from childhood and the "concordance" with the paternal character traits with which we endow this "great man" do not in fact seem to suffice in this case.

Hatred and Interdiction

In all the texts in which Freud tackles group psychology, the putting into action of "psychic reality" within "material reality" is the decisive element of the potential translation of the individual to the socius. Thus in "Thoughts for the Times on the War and Death": the brutal transport of psychic reality into the reality of war is due to the fact that from the beginning man as killer never ceased inhabiting civilized man, the drive satisfaction of the former obfuscating the latter's use of judgment. As descendants of an infinitely long line of murderers,[37] our excitation at the idea of war brims over the constraint of morality and reveals the source of man's inflexible attraction to killing.

The invention of psychoanalysis, the discovery of psychic reality, and the question of murder are in truth contemporaneous. The reference to Oedipus the King in the letter to Fließ of September 21, 1897 demonstrates this and describes the power of the relation between fantasy and the achievement in act of the double crime – killing the father, sexually possessing the mother – with the reversal of the punishment against oneself. Between murder, guilt, and renunciation, Freud thus from the first seeks out an origin of the civilizing process. An origin capable of knotting together individual morality and collective ethics. An origin which he will place within the trajectory of an inaugural act, its effacement and the cultural attempt at holding back its return. This is where Freud draws his initial conception of the social alliance: when the murder of the primal father – a figure intensely beloved for his potency and protection, and furiously hated for this very potency and his limitless power – leads to the mutual dependence of a fraternal pact in which are rooted renunciations, atonements, and totemic prohibitions under the order of the "conscience-morality-taboo."

There can be no doubt that the introduction of narcissism and the death drive led to profound modifications. From the interiorizing of the tutelary figure to the especially proximate relationship between the id and the superego, we see how little by little "omniscience of the superego" (*Allwissenheit des Überichs*),[38] the direct heir of the id, cares nothing for the difference between the consequences of the actual execution of the act and the anxiety faced with the internal authority when the act is carried out only by the intentionality of thinking. However what undoubtedly affects most profoundly the "economy" of guilt is the fact that the moral conscience, the product of the reversal of the aggression toward the inside, finds its source in the death drive itself. This leads Freud, speaking to Einstein, to call his theory a "heresy" (*Ketzerei*).[39] Did Freud at this time already have some foresight of the ravage to come and the effects of the "perfection of instruments"[40] – an expression used in their epistolary exchange of 1932? Was he contemplating a novel version of the wreck? Had he already conceived, in his own way, what Adorno would call "absolute negativity" – absolute because the act of extermination has no backside, no hideout, no handling of stolen goods?[41]

There can be no doubt that in *The Man Moses*, "the tragedy of the primal father" is at once united with the hatred against the Jewish people and the founding act of monotheism. It speaks another standard in order to consider the horror. Not because the sense of guilt passed on immemorably, generation after generation, would, in the anti-Semitic hatred of the time, come up against the monstrous endpoint of its expiation.[42] But because suddenly the probable elimination of the Jews reveals to the West how it hates unfailingly, just as immemorably as the transmission, something of itself: not something outside it, but something inside it, the very core of its civilization, simultaneously the origin of culture and the genealogy of the mind.[43] It is thus not a matter of a cultures affair (in the plural). It concerns the West's self-hatred, which demolishes the very soul of the cultural task. With *The Man Moses*, we consequently find ourselves in the paradoxical situation in which, when mass murder is on the brink of finding the verbal logic of its methodical practice, Freud becomes the latest narrator of a story dominated by the examination of the birth of a people and its law (*loi*), and implicitly with the threat of its disappearance.

In this sense, even if Freud relates the postulates of *The Man Moses* to *Totem and Taboo*, even if in both cases Freud suggests solutions permitting the id wronged in its demand for satisfaction to compensate itself for the loss, the settlements between renunciation and compensation are not at all identical in each case. What comparison between the epic recounting the crime, such as it is presented in *Totem and Taboo*, and that which Freud describes concerning the foundation of a people in which the murder of Moses, its burying and its return, define the position of a lawgiver? This is a serious point since in this case the historicizing of the figure of the "great man" and the treatment of the fault leads not to a theogony but to ethical legislation.

Bruno Karsenti, in *Moses and the Idea of a People*, convincingly points out the difference between the anthropological dimension of *Totem and Taboo* and the political dimension of *Moses*. Whereas the ambivalence of the totemic clan with regard to the father is perceptible in the very act of the sacrifice (which simultaneously repeats through hallucination the leveling of the father and his triumph), the consuming of the sacrificial animal constitutes in itself a compensation. By partaking in the meal, the divinity guarantees the identificatory transaction alongside the sacrifice offering the father "satisfaction […] for the outrage inflicted on him in the same act in which that deed is commemorated."[44] Remembrance takes the form of a festival, a moment of intense excitation rooted in sensorality.

Is this excitation missing in the case of Jewish monotheism? The intoxication of the moral asceticism which moves these "great ascetics," the observance of the ethic bordering on the "grandiose" and the unfathomable,[45] the insatiable sense of guilt, over-abstraction, over-impersonalization stricken with the mark of ideality argue in favor of decreased excitation. On the contrary, all indicate the persistence of the grandiose character of the parental agency whose superego is the heir. This grandiose about which Freud argues in *Group Psychology and the Analysis of the Ego* which, produced out of the introjection of the parental agency, is also the heir of the narcissistic self cathexis by the child: the subject benefits from being able to identify with the traits that the parental figure admires in him. In the form of ascetic ideality there thus returns in secret the submission to the grandiose father whom it is still a matter of satisfying – the vibration of the ascetic finding material for compensation for all the renunciations.

Despite all that has been said, this does not solve the problem of the transition of the individual to the socius. As a matter of fact, not only the procurement by the child of supplemental love – emerged out of the drive sacrifice made by the ego to the superego – has no strictly social equivalent. But above all, even if "the great man is precisely the authority for whose sake the achievement is carried out" and so in this way "in group psychology the role of the superego falls to him,"[46] it is not nevertheless possible to specify the authority which provides the norm of what should be judged higher. In the case of the victory of paternal law ("*droit*"), continues Freud, "It cannot in this case be the father, since he is only elevated into being an authority by the advance itself."[47] Shortly before, Freud noted, "[…] we must recall that the father too was once a child."[48] This remark, which explains the chronological going-back to the initial founder, Akhenaton, in any case undermines the simplicity of the transition. To be sure, the child has a father who is the bearer of authority and the shared norm. But how did the norm shared by the community shape itself?

The "Law" (*droit*) in Quotation Marks

Here Freud is entangled in three lines of thought: first, the specifically ahistorical process of the inscription of memory traces; second, historical time related to the successive transformations of civilizations; and lastly the burden of contemporaneous events. We find an initial trace of them in *Civilization and Its Discontents* when he decides to put the word "law" ("*droit*") in quotation marks. Communal life admittedly becomes possible only when a plurality of individuals manages to constitute a more powerful grouping than each of its members since it is by this means that the power of the community counters, as "law" ("*droit*"), each individual's violence. But this "decisive step of civilization," which leads to the exigency of justice, in fact says nothing, writes Freud, "as to the ethical value of such a law (*Recht*)."[49] We merely observe that it "seems" (Freud's word) to be a right which everyone has contributed to and from which all benefit. Two years later, in "Why War?," he will ask Einstein to "replace the word 'might' by the balder and harsher word 'violence,'"[50] considering that the organs created to keep watch over the observance of the laws (*lois*) have but themselves to execute "legal acts of violence."[51] This conception is perhaps close to "legitimate violence" developed by Weber in 1919 but whose value would have radically changed in 1933: the main preoccupation of each party in the dialogue is to know what will become of law (*droit*) under the Nazi regime's iron rule.

The declared anti-Semitism of a jurist as renowned as Carl Schmitt, his fidelity to Roman Catholicism, his extremely violent indictment against the Jewish conception of the law (*loi*), and his deep-seated hostility to the Weimer republic coupled with a conception of order by way of dictatorial sovereignty all function as the early warning signs of the undertaking-to-come of the "de-Judaization" of the *law* (*Gesetz*) for the benefit of the new German law (*Recht*). Schmitt – who enthusiastically comments on Hitler's speech on the state given in 1933 and 1934,[52] but in particular concludes the 1936 Congress on "Judaism in the Science of Law (*droit*)" with an address, "The German Science of Law (*droit*) in its Struggle against the Jewish Spirit" – is one of its major artisans. There notably figures in this speech the justification for the "purging of the libraries"[53] thanks to which one may fight against "the Jewish spirit" of the *law* (*loi*) which – condemned for its abstract rationalism, "the empty legality of [its] false neutrality,"[54] and its reference to the norm – must make way for the living concreteness of an instinctual *law* (*droit*) inspired by nature.

Thus when Freud undertakes the writing of *The Man Moses*, "the purification of legal literature"[55] is advancing at the same pace as the public burning of books. This is the context in which Thomas Mann joins up with him, seeing him as the Goethe of modernity, a particularly damaged modernity since the Goethean "demonic" and the "drive quality" bequeathed by the Romantics have become the weapon in the hands of the Nazis thanks to which must be "broken the primacy of reason, and restored in triumph, in their primitive vital law (*droit*), the forces of darkness and the abyssal depths, the instinctive and the irrational."[56] Freud will specify in the postscript to the *Autobiographical Study* that receiving the Goethe Prize was "the climax of my life as a citizen. Soon afterwards the boundaries of our country narrowed and the nation would know no more of us."[57]

Narrowing and ostracism: how may we relate repetition to the force of missing memories when, on the one hand, a *Führer* proclaims his power to restore the German people to its unity by instituting supremacy and, on the other, another *Führer* was at the root of the ethics and commandments of God to which he himself was subject?

Moses Created the Jews

"Faced with the new persecutions, one asks oneself again how the Jews have come to what they are and why they have attracted this underlying hatred," Freud writes to Arnold Zweig on September 30, 1934. "I soon discovered the formula: Moses created the Jews. So I gave my work the title: *The Man Moses, A Historical Novel*."[58] Which Freud repeats in this very work: "And since we know that behind the God who had chosen the Jews and freed them from Egypt stands the figure of Moses, who had done precisely that, ostensibly at God's command, we venture to declare that it was this one man Moses who created the Jews."[59] In the meantime, he still wrote to Eitingon on November 13, 1934: "I am no good at historical romances. Let us leave them to Thomas Mann."[60] He then decided to establish his research on scientific grounds.

But why Thomas Mann? Because the "novelist" had just completed, in 1933, the first two volumes of *Joseph and His Brothers* (*The Stories of Jacob* and *Young Joseph*) and he was readying to set historically the third story of his tetralogy, *Joseph in Egypt*, in the Amarna period during the reign of Akhenaton. At the time Mann had in no way considered writing the novella, *The Tables of the Law* (*Das Gesetz*).[61] It was written during his exile in the United States in 1942 at the request of Armin L. Robinson just before he began writing *Doctor Faustus*. The project, *The Ten Commandments: Ten Short Novels of Hitler's War against the Moral Code*, directly concerns the violations committed by the *Führer*. But for Thomas Mann, this *Führer* was the unconscious aspect of German genius: a counter-artist (*Gegenkünstler*[62]) who seeks to shape the German people in accordance with the key elements of this new law (*droit*), the "lout" of the figure of the "great man."

There is consequently nothing random in the fact that Thomas Mann presents his Moses in the desert receiving the tables of the law from God as the artist shaping the primal matter of this group of desert wanderers much like a sculptor, giving shape to their "formless souls" (p. 17). Without doubt his clipped speech differs from the "drawling, fluent discourse" (p. 27) of Aaron. But there is no doubt, one would like to add, that he is wholly contrary to Hitler's rants. Pleasure in instructing is at the heart of Moses's enthusiasm. Not that he is spared by the complaints, indeed the hatred of the crowd and its about-faces against the exodus and the covenant (p. 48). Nevertheless, he perseveres, he carries on "chisel[ling] and chip[ping] away" at the "raw material of flesh and blood" (p. 67). And he does justice before installing the judges teaching the law (p. 64). This "justice," writes Mann, "was directly connected to and protected by the invisibility of God" (p. 61), for out of this invisibility emanated the very activity of thought, the refusal of chaos, the requirement of distinctions in all – and these concerned every aspect of life, from the burial of excrements to alimentary prohibitions and all forms of defilement. Pure and impure, pride and aversion (p. 68): thus there was imposed the need to set and keep, carved in the stone of His mountain, the formula of the commandments to be respected, the divine moral law (*loi*) which Moses brought to his uneducated, wavering people (p. 83).

Assmann is quite right when he qualifies *The Tables of the Law* as an "antifascist manifesto."[63] At its center is placed the object par excellence of Nazi hatred: judicial abstraction and the functioning of autonomous categories independent of subjectivity. What is more, the stature of the lawgiver reveals itself there as the precise opposite of the figure of the "great hypnotist," the all-powerful leader described in *Group Psychology and the Analysis of the Ego*. Quite the contrary, Moses's struggle is human and onerous whereas the return of the formless, of which the worshipping of the golden calf is the emblem, looms. We want images, we want gods to worship just like other peoples, proclaims the crowd "celebrating their miserable freedom" (p. 96) while Moses on Sinai invents the consonant alphabet allowing him to "to write the words of everyday language of every people" (pp. 90–91) and to forge thereby the very principle of universalism – that of God, that of language, that of the law (*loi*) – , carving in the rock the letters of the Ten Commandments which he stains with his own blood (p. 93). But the blood of this judicial core is not the soil of "Blut und Boden," of "Blood and Soil." It is not the swell of "black stupidity" (p. 104) spread by a brute sitting on a golden throne. In this civilizing heroic novel, it possesses the force of a symbol at the very time "the final solution" is decided on. That is, at the time when Germany is destroying itself by means of the actual realization of the fantasmatic dogma of its purity.

No, Freud could not imagine that Thomas Mann would write *The Tables of the Law*. Yet it is his rectitude that he honors in 1935 when he wished the novelist all the best upon his sixtieth birthday:

> In the name of a countless number of your contemporaries I can express to you our confidence that you will never do or say – for an author's words are deeds – anything that is cowardly or base. Even in times and circumstances that perplex the judgement you will take the right path and point it out to others.[64]

Together with the Zurich publisher Emil Oprecht, in whose city he had taken refuge at the time, Thomas Mann will found a journal, *Mass und Wert*, whose "anti-barbarism" program aimed at condemning "the euphoria" of belief. The year before, on February 27, 1934, Gustav Bally published a far-reaching article in the *Neue Zürcher Zeitung* asking Jung to clarify his position just as he had taken charge of the new *Zentralblatt* – or more precisely of the *Journal for Psychotherapy and Its Bordering Fields, including Medical Psychology and Psychic Hygiene*. And "psychic hygiene" resonates here with all the violence of the hygienist policy of "Blut und Boden." In its pages he published an editorial, never to be forgotten, celebrating the creative force and sparks of the Aryan unconscious, apt to develop new cultural forms – whereas the Jew, "relatively nomad," could never succeed at producing a proper cultural form. Jung thus develops the idea that the Jewish categories of psychology, devised by a Freud who had no knowledge of the German soul, treats these representative creative forms like a "banal simplistic swamp." And he declares that "the Aryan unconscious has a higher potential than the Jewish unconscious."[65] Worse still, in 1936, Jung writes his essay on Wotan in which he shows the extent of the Nazi involvement in his theory of archetypes.

What did Freud sense in 1914 when he contested Jung's archetypes and broke with him in writing *Totem and Taboo*? In fact, in making Wotan one of the mythic hearts of the Germanic unconscious and Hitler the "prophet" of its howling vortex, capable of gathering the herd together emotionally,[66] he spared himself from questioning the root of the mass's folly. Jung moreover wrote: "Despite their crankiness, the Wotan-worshippers seem to have judged things more accurately than the worshippers of reason. Apparently everyone had forgotten that Wotan is a Germanic datum of first importance, the truest expression and unsurpassed personification of a fundamental quality that is particularly characteristic of the Germans."[67] Thus old Wotan, the autonomous German archetype whose unconscious influence took hold of the individual human being, greater explains National Socialism than the three rational factors which are psychology, economics, and political science.[68]

The incriminated psychology is without doubt Freud's, thrown into the same basket as the economic and political analyses devised by liberals or Marxists. But is it perhaps more specifically that promoted by Freud starting from the first of the three essays in *The Man Moses and Monotheistic Religion*? Moses versus Wotan? This would be another version of the violence, which Heine had long ago shown as likely,[69] generated by the confusion between energetics, culture, and politics. This amalgam, promoted by the new version of scientific thought – the naturalness of the race – is effectively in the process of obtaining the "mystical" support of the people. Now for Jung – but Freud had already highlighted this in *Group Psychology and the Analysis of the Ego* when he emphasized the "mystical" character of the hypnotic phenomenon[70] – this mystical character is the very mark of Hitler. "Take the very name of the Nazi State. They call it the Third Reich. Why?" Because the First Reich was the German Holy Roman Empire and the Second was that founded by Bismarck. But there is a deeper, mystical significance, too, continues Jung: "to every German the expression 'Third Reich' brings echoes in his unconscious of the Biblical hierarchy. Thus Hitler, who more than once has indicated he is aware of his mystic calling, appears to the devotees of the Third Reich as something more than mere man."[71] And he concludes: "Hitler's power is not political; it is *magic*."[72]

This was why he had to lend his credibility to the law (*loi*) against magic, against the mystical of the masses, and against the excitation of any election whatsoever. In order to do this, the promotion of morality had to be a specifically human legislative endeavor, that is, fragile, and subject to be dealt a death-blow. Wide room had to be made for murder, including in Jewish memory. The veils of forgetting had to be stripped away from it and its effect – repression, return, legislated interdictions – re-implanted in the unsteady matter of civilizations by separating them from any appropriation by a given dogma. By seizing upon Moses, Freud no doubt also had in mind the secular simulacrum of the *Führer*, Hitler, and his parodic call for Nazi "political dogma" as well as loyalty and faith.[73] Bringing to light their shared roots – an indifference to reality twinned with psychotic delirium – meant taking a final step toward the secularization of thinking by turning, in Freud's eyes, Scripture into the true legacy of the Jewish tradition. In short, at that moment there "probably" remained a single hope for the "gang of killers"[74] that we are: well beyond the causes of the persecution of the Jews accused of being Christ's killers,[75] the "phylogenetic" achievements of our morality must not be consumed by savagery and what is best in monotheism – the advancement of the life of the mind – outlives the dark times.

Notes

* Translated from French by Steven Jaron.

1 A literal rendering of Freud's German title is given for reasons the author discusses in footnote 4. (Translator's note.)

2 See E. J. Rolnik (2012), *Freud in Zion: Psychoanalysis and the Making of Modern Jewish Identity* (London, Karnac), pp. 65–66.

3 The author uses the French for "law," *droit*, here whereas in the essay's subtitle she uses *loi*, also translated into English as "law." French, like German, has two distinct words for "law" – *loi/Gesestz* and *droit/Recht*, translated literally as "right" but colloquially as "law" – whereas English has but a single term, "law." Broadly speaking, the former refers to more general, underlying judicial principles while the latter refers to specific statutes or acts. In order to maintain this distinction, where necessary the author's French and/or German is retained in parentheses. (Translator's note.)

4 The translation of the essay's title in English (*Moses and Monotheism*) omits the presence of "the man" in the German title, *Der Mann Moses und die monotheistische Religion*.

5 S. Freud (1930), *Das Unbehagen in der Kultur*, *GW* 14, p. 481.

6 Ibid., p. 505.

7 Ibid., p. 481.

8 A postulate which Darwin vigorously criticized. See L. Ritvo (1990), *Darwin's Influence on Freud: A Tale of Two Sciences* (New Haven and London, Yale University Press).

9 Hegel, *Reason in History*; and the commentary of P. Ricœur (1985) *Temps et récit* [Time and Narrative] volume 3, *Le temps raconté* [Time Recounted] (Paris, Le Seuil), p. 289.
10 Cf. A Kojève (1979), "L'idée de la mort dans la philosophie de Hegel" [The Ideas of Death in Hegel's Philosophy], *Introduction à la lecture de Hegel* [Introduction to a Reading of Hegel] (Paris, Gallimard), pp. 529–575.
11 S. Freud (1930), *Das Unbehagen in der Kultur*, *GW* 14, p. 501 f.; *Civilization and Its Discontents*, *SE* 21, p. 141.
12 Ibid., *GW* 14, p. 502; *SE* 21, p. 141.
13 S. Freud (1927), *Zukunkft einer Illusion*, *GW* 14, p. 369; *The Future of an Illusion*, *SE* 21, p. 46.
14 Ibid., *GW* 14, p. 374; *SE* 21, p. 51.
15 S. Freud (1932), "Why War?," *SE* 22, p. 213.
16 S. Freud (1940), *Abriss der Psychoanalyse*, *GW* 17, pp. 112–113; *An Outline of Psychoanalysis*, *SE* 23, p. 206. See also S. Freud (1905), *Drei Abhandlungen zur Sexualtheorie*, *GW* 5, p. 78; *Three Essays on the Theory of Sexuality*, *SE* 7, pp. 177–178.
17 S. Freud (1913), "Das Interesse an der Psychoanalyse," *GW* 8, pp. 418–419; "The Claims of Psychoanalysis to Scientific Interest," *SE* 13, p. 188.
18 S. Freud (1912), "Schlußwork der Onanie-diskussion," *GW* 8, p. 337; "Contributions to a Discussion on Masturbation," *SE* 12, p. 248.
19 S. Freud (1939) *Der Mann Moses und die monotheistische Religion: Drei Abhandlungen*, *GW* 16, p. 115; *The Man Moses and Monotheistic Religion: Three Essays*, *SE* 23, p. 17.
20 Y. H. Yerushalmi (1991), *Freud's Moses: Judaism Terminable and Interminable* (New Haven and London, Yale University Press) p. 17.
21 Ibid.
22 Note that from beginning to end in *The Man Moses*, the "great man" is called *Führer*, an ordinary term also used in the first German language translations of Rousseau's *Social Contract* to indicate "leader."
23 C. Bonomi (2015), *The Cut and the Building of Psychoanalysis (Volume 1): Sigmund Freud and Emma Eckstein* (Hove and New York, Routledge), pp. 3–4.
24 H. Arendt (1953), "Religion and Politics," in *Essays in Understanding, 1930–1954: Formation, Exile, and Totalitarianism*, Jerome Kohn (editor and introduction) (New York, Schocken, 1994), p. 383. First published in *Confluence* 2, 3, 1953.
25 S. Freud (1939), *Der Mann Moses*, *GW* 16, p. 156; *The Man Moses*, *SE* 23, p. 54. Translation modified.
26 S. Freud (1935), *Nachschrift zur "Selbstdarstellung,"* *GW* 16, p. 33; postscript to *An Autobiographical Study*, *SE* 20, p. 72.
27 S. Freud (1939), *Der Mann Moses*, *GW* 16, p. 113; *The Man Moses*, *SE* 23, p. 16.
28 M. Bloch (1949), *Apologie pour l'histoire ou Métier d'historien* [Apology for History or the Trade of Historian] (Paris, Armand Colin, 1997), p. 157.
29 L. Febvre (1953), *Combats pour l'histoire* [Struggles for History] (Paris, Armand Colin), p. 23.
30 S. Freud (1937), "Konstruktionen in der Analyse," *GW* 16, p. 55; "Constructions in Analysis," *SE* 23, p. 268.
31 Ibid., *GW* 16, p. 56; *SE* 23, p. 269. Emphasis in the original.
32 S. Freud (1939), *Der Mann Moses*, *GW* 16, p. 190; *The Man Moses*, *SE* 23, p. 85.

33 Y. H. Yerushalmi (1991), *Freud's Moses: Judaism Terminable and Interminable* (New Haven and London, Yale University Press), p. 31.
34 S. Freud (1933), *Neue Folge der Vorlesungen zur Einführung in die Psychoanalyse, GW* 15, p. 181; *New Introductory Lectures on Psychoanalysis, SE* 22, p. 168.
35 Ibid.
36 S. Freud (1939), *Der Mann Moses,GW*16, p. 216; *The Man Moses, SE* 23, p. 109.
37 S. Freud (1915) *Zeitgemäßes über Krieg und Tod, GW* 10, p. 350.
38 S. Freud (1930), *Das Unbehagen in der Kultur, GW* 16, p. 497; *Civilization and Its Discontents, SE* 21, p. 131.
39 S. Freud (1933), "Warum Krieg?," *GW*, 16, p. 22; "Why War?," *SE* 22, p. 210.
40 Ibid., *SE* 22, p. 212.
41 See T. W. Adorno's remarks (1966) in the "After Auschwitz" section of *Negative Dialektik* [Negative Dialectics] (Frankfurt, Suhrkamp). See also T. W. Adorno (1951), *Minima Moralia: Reflexionen aus dem Beschædigten Leben* [Minima Moralia: Reflections from Damaged Life] (Frankfurt, Suhrkamp).
42 S. Freud (1939), *Der Mann Moses,GW* 16, p. 246; *The Man Moses, SE* 23, p. 136: "In a certain sense they have in that way taken a tragic load of guilt on themselves; they have been made to pay heavy penance for it."
43 I'm referring to the work of P. Lacoue-Labarthe (1987), *La Fiction du politique: Heidegger, l'art et la politique* [The Fiction of Policy: Heidegger, Art, and Politics] (Paris, Christian Bourgois), notably pp. 58–81.
44 S. Freud (1913), *Totem und Tabu GW* 9, pp. 180–181; *Totem and Taboo, SE* 13, p. 150.
45 S. Freud (1939), *Der Mann Moses, GW* 16, p. 230; *The Man Moses, SE* 23, p. 122.
46 S. Freud (1939), *Der Mann Moses, GW* 16, p. 225; *The Man Moses, SE* 23, p. 117.
47 S. Freud (1939), *Der Mann Moses, GW* 16, p. 225; *The Man Moses, SE* 23, p. 118.
48 S. Freud (1939), *Der Mann Moses,GW* 16, p. 218; *The Man Moses, SE* 23, p. 110.
49 S. Freud (1930), *Das Unbehagen in der Kultur, GW* 14, p. 455; *Civilization and Its Discontents, SE* 21, p. 95.
50 S. Freud (1932), "Warum Krieg?," *GW* 16, p. 14; "Why War?," *SE* 22, pp. 203–204.
51 Ibid., *GW*, 16, p. 16; *SE* 22, p. 205.
52 C. Schmitt, "Le Führer protège le droit. À propos du discours d'Adolf Hitler au Reichstag du 13 juillet 1934" [The Führer Protects the Law: Concerning Adolf Hitler's Speech to the Reichstag on July 13, 1934], *Cités* 14, 2, 2003, pp. 165–171.
53 C. Schmitt, "La science allemande du droit dans sa lutte contre l'esprit juif" [The German Science of Law in Its Struggle Against the Jewish Spirit], *Cités* 14, 2, 2003, pp. 173–180; here p. 174.
54 C. Schmitt, "Le Führer protège le droit. À propos du discours d'Adolf Hitler au Reichstag du 13 juillet 1934," *Cités* 14, 2, 2003, p. 165.
55 C. Schmitt, "La science allemande du droit dans sa lutte contre l'esprit juif,' *Cités* 14, 2, 2003, p. 175.
56 T. Mann (1933), "Freud's Position in the History of Modern Thought," H.T. Lowe-Porter (translator), *The Criterion: A Literary Review* 12, pp. 549–570; and T. Mann (1936), "Freud and the Future," *The International Journal of Psychoanalysis* 37, 1956, pp. 106–115.
57 S. Freud (1935), *Nachschrift zur "Selbstdarstellung," GW* 16, p. 33; postscript to *An Autobiographical Study, SE* 20, p. 73.
58 *The Letters of Sigmund Freud and Arnold Zweig* (1970), E. L. Freud (editor), E. & W. Robson-Scott (translators) (New York, Harcourt, Brace and World), p. 91.

59 S. Freud (1939), *Der Mann Moses*, *GW* 16, p. 213; *The Man Moses*, *SE* 23, p. 106.
60 Quoted in E. Jones (1957), *The Life and Work of Sigmund Freud, 1919–1939: The Last Phase*, volume 3 (New York, Basic Books), p. 194.
61 T. Mann (1943), *The Tables of the Law*, Marion Faber & Stephen Lehmann (translators); Michael Wood (afterword) (London, Haus Publishing, 2010).
62 T. Mann (1984), entry of July 7, 1938 in *Diaries, 1918–1939* (Seattle, Thrift Books), p. 303.
63 J. Assmann (2015), "Mose gegen Hitler: Die zehn Gebote als antifaschistes Manifest" [Moses against Hitler: The Ten Commandments as Antifascist Manifesto], *Thomas Mann Jahrbuch*, volume 28, pp. 47–61.
64 S. Freud (1935), "Thomas Mann zum 60. Gerburtstag," *GW* 16, p. 249; "To Thomas Mann on His Sixtieth Birthday," *SE* 22, p. 255.
65 C. G. Jung (1934), "Zur gegenwärtigen Lage der Psychotherapie" [On the Present Position of Psychotherapy], *Zivilisation im Übergang, Gesammelte Werke*, volume 10 (Walter-Verlag, Olten, Switzerland, 1974), pp. 190–191, published in 1934 in the *Zentralblatt für Psychotherapie und ihrer Grenzgebiete einschlie ßlich der Medizinischen Psychologie und Psychischen Hygiene*, volume 7, pp. 1–16 (consulted on archiv.org).
66 C. G. Jung (1938), "Diagnosing the Dictators," in *C.G. Jung Speaking: Interviews and Encounters*, W. McGuire & R.F.C. Hull (editors) (Princeton, Princeton University Press, 1977), p. 118.
67 C. G. Jung (1936), "Wotan," *Neue Schweizer Rundschau*, March 1936; republished in *Zivilisation im Übergang, Gesammelte Werke*, volume 10, pp. 203–218 (here, p. 209); and in C. G, Jung (1958), *Essays on Contemporary Events*, Barbara Hannah (translator) & R. F. C. Hull (editor) (London and New York, Routledge, 2002), p. 19.
68 Ibid.
69 H. Heine (1834), *On the History of Religion and Philosophy in Germany* (Cambridge University Press, Cambridge, 2007), p. 116: "A play will be enacted in Germany which will make the French Revolution look like a harmless idyll. It is still rather silent, to be sure; and if someone or other is making a bit of noise now, do not think that these are the true actors. They are only small dogs running around in the empty arena, barking and snapping at each other until the hour comes when the troop of gladiators will arrive to fight to the death."
70 S. Freud (1921), *Massenpsychologie und Ich-Analyse*, *GW* 13, p. 127; *Group Psychology and the Analysis of the Ego*, *SE* 18, p. 115.
71 C. G. Jung (1938), "Diagnosing the Dictators," in *C.G. Jung Speaking: Interviews and Encounters*,W. McGuire & R. F. C. Hull (editors) (Princeton, Princeton University Press, 1977), pp. 117–118.
72 Ibid., p. 118. Emphasis in the original.
73 This is what is found throughout *Mein Kampf*. See for instance Adolf Hitler (1925/1927), *Mein Kampf*, two volumes in one (München 1944), pp. 50, 418, 423.
74 S. Freud (1915), *Zeitgemäßes über Krieg und Tod*, *GW* 10, p. 351 ("eine Rotte von Mördern").
75 On this point, see R. Loewenstein (1952), *Psychanalyse de l'antisémitisme* [Psychoanalysis of Antisemitism] (Paris, Presses universitaires de France, 2001), p. 83.

Editor's Introduction to Chapter 4

Lawrence J. Brown

Merav Roth creatively imagines Moses and Freud as "literary twins": just as Moses has received the Torah from God and is charged with fostering and protecting its teachings, so Freud has created psychoanalysis as an equivalent body of secular teachings. Roth, who has previously written about the connection between the author and the reader, suggests that *Moses and Monotheism* served a dual role for the elderly Freud that "enables him to perform his 'art of mourning' both as a writer (Ogden, 2000) and as a reader (Roth, 2020)." Roth further develops the theme of many dualities which run through *Moses and Monotheism*: Moses and Akhenaten as the two Egyptian founders of monotheistic religion; two 'characters' in this story who are both named Moses; two Gods who are later subsumed into one monotheistic God, just to name several of these dyads. Roth skillfully discusses the subtle differences between these dualisms and how the knitting together of the more ancient Israelite beliefs of the slaves freed in Exodus with a later group of Jews who had not been part of the original migration. Roth appears to suggest that Freud himself may have had some doubts regarding these dualities and references Dorfman's (2020) ironic observation that "although Freud speaks of two figures of Moses and of two Jewish gods, nowhere in his book does he mention the word 'double'" (p. 183).

Roth also takes us into her area of expertise, the notion of a 'transference twin' in which the reader forms an identification with the author, and she elucidates the different types of literary twins which appear in *Moses and Monotheism*. Her view of Freud and Moses as literary twins deepens our appreciation of their respective contributions to the collective literature of mankind that deals with the wish for a paradise and the recognition of reality. Freud's desire to remain in his beloved Austria, and most assuredly continue his writings, was crushed by the reality of the Nazi Anschluss from which he barely escaped. Similarly, Moses' expectation to enter the Promised Land along with the Exodus of former Israelite slaves he had freed, was halted by God on Mount Nebo when he said to Moses

DOI: 10.4324/9781003272045-8

that he would not be entering the Holy Land. Freud had long worried that his professional fate would be that of Moses and "he feared that the price of his triumph might be his own death" (Anzieu, p. 186). Dr. Roth's chapter is a valued contribution to the notion of "literary twins" and her discussion of Freud and Moses deepens our understanding of this twinship.

4 "Moses – Freud's Literary Twin"

Merav Roth

Introduction – Why Moses?

This chapter delves into a reading of Freud's *Moses and Monotheism* (1939) from an interdisciplinary perspective of literature and psychoanalysis. It explores the way Freud, as he approached the end of his life, used Moses as a literary twin, whose story offered Freud a rich and complex perspective on his journey as a leader and a prophet, and helped him to work – through various aspects of his path.

The role of the literary character is to offer the reader an opportunity to work through his inner aspirations, anxieties, and unconscious phantasies in the special terms of literary reading that I have elsewhere termed "The distancing paradox" (Roth, 2020, pp. 33–39). When the reader is distancing to the far-away place and time of the story, characterized by foreign traits of the hero, foreign habits, language, costumes, and customs, it paradoxically enables him to come closer to himself. The literary hero appears to be so far and different from the reader that he unconsciously lets go of his defenses and identifies deeply with the story, without realizing that by doing so he is actually working through his own story.

Freud's reconstruction of the story of Moses is not only an historical account, but also a creative reading of it, as reflected in his subsequently added subtitle 'A historical novel' (Rolnik, p. 133). The literary hero Moses is the leader of a nation, who regards his Torah (his biblical doctrine) as the holy Torah, the only Torah, a Torah which is named after him (Moses' Torah) and endures long after his death. Moses passionately believes that it will enlighten his disciples and free them through their encounter with the supreme truth. The conviction that this Torah was handed to Moses by God, endows it with greatness and high importance. I suggest that this protagonist offers a mirror image to Freud's aspirations that his psychoanalytic Torah has the power to free those who 'believe in it' and lead them to a higher intellectual level of sublimation and supreme truth. Moreover, that it will grant Freud himself eternal existence such as that of his literary hero Moses. At the same time – Moses' failures and misfortunes

DOI: 10.4324/9781003272045-9

offer Freud an opportunity to investigate and mourn his own unresolved conflicts and struggles and repair his wounds.

Moses and Monotheism– a Story of Doubles

Moses and Monotheism was Freud's final original work, and many see it as his heritage and will (See for instance Yerushalmi, 1991; Derrida, 1996; Bernstein, 1998). Although it had earlier versions, it was finally published in its full version in 1939, when death was viewed through Freud's bedroom window. Yet we know it was by no means the beginning of his interest in the figure of Moses, with whom he was already intensely preoccupied many years earlier, as evident in his fascinating text about Michelangelo's sculpture of Moses (1914). In "The Moses of Michelangelo" (1914), Freud portrays Moses in the following words: "the giant frame with its tremendous physical power becomes only a concrete expression of the highest mental achievement that is possible in a man, that of struggling successfully against an inward passion for the sake of a cause to which he has devoted himself " (Freud, 1914, p. 233). We could think of "The Moses of Michelangelo" as a portrait that sheds light on the younger Freud, whereas *Moses and Monotheism* (1939) could be seen as Freud's "portrait of old man."[1] Eduard Said (2003), claims that it is even written in a unique late style (spätstil) characteristic of the final works of writers. Freud was finalizing this work in a foreign country, only a year after his "exodus from Egypt," i.e. the traumatic deportation from his beloved motherland to London due to the Nazi invasion of Austria, suffering from cancer and old age, undoubtedly realizing that this text would become his swan song. This adds to the text tremendous weight and significance (see also Said, 2003; Dorfman, 2020). At various times in the past Freud turned to literature,[2] when looking for ways to articulate traumatic, uncanny, "unclaimed experiences" (Caruth, 1996). Caruth, who saw *Moses and Monotheism* as Freud's late elaboration on his theory of trauma, wrote: "If Freud turns to literature to describe traumatic experience, it is because literature, like psychoanalysis, is interested in the complex relation between knowing and not knowing. And it is at the specific point at which knowing and not knowing intersect that the language of literature and the psychoanalytic theory of traumatic experience precisely meet" (Caruth, 1996, pp. 2–3).

In *Moses and Monotheism*, Freud re-read the traditional account of Moses in light of new archeological findings at Tel-El-Amarna. If we read Moses' story as a literary work, we find that the thesis offered by Freud-the-reader reveals multiple literary twins or doubles. I shall try to trace their role and introduce the idea that they represent different aspects that help Freud in this fragile moment of existence. I suggest that his reading in *Moses and Monotheism* enabled him to perform his "art of mourning" both as a writer (Ogden, 2000) and as a reader (Roth, 2020), working through and coming to terms not only with the finitude of his personal life but also with the limits of psychoanalysis and the fate of his legacy.

Let us first be reminded of the reconstruction offered by Freud, while paying attention to the various doubles that play a part in it. As we will soon discover, we are introduced to a few literary twins in the story as well as between Freud-the-reader and the story's characters. It appears in Freud's words at the end of the second part of *Moses and Monotheism* named "If Freud was an Egyptian": "Our findings may be thus expressed in the most concise formula. Jewish history is familiar to us for its dualities: two groups of people who came together to form the nation, two kingdoms into which this nation split, two gods' names in the documentary sources of the Bible. To these we add two fresh ones: the foundation of two religions – the first repressed by the second but nevertheless later emerging victoriously behind it, and two religious founders, who are both called by the same name of Moses and whose personalities we have to distinguish from each other. All of these dualities are the necessary consequences of the first one: the fact that one portion of the people had an experience which must be regarded as traumatic and which the other portion escaped." (Freud, 1939, p. 52). We read that there were **two** Egyptian leaders who introduced monotheism to **two** national groups (Akhenaten to the Egyptians and Moses to the Hebrews); **two** Moses and **two** Gods. There were even **two** writings by Freud regarding the same course of events told in **two** formats – that of Totem and Taboo (1913) and again in *Moses and Monotheism* (1939).[3]

According to Freud's interpretation of the new archeological findings and some readings of the history of the Hebrew people (especially by Meyer and Sellin), Freud, the father of psychoanalysis, suggested that Moses, the father of the Jewish religion, was actually an Egyptian, and that he was not the one who invented monotheism. Monotheism was introduced for the first time in history by the pharaoh Akhenaten. "Becoming monotheist, Akhenaten tried to cancel the multiplicity of his dynasty (Amenhotep I, II, III, IV)" (Dorfman, 2020, p. 186) by taking upon himself his unique name and path. "But if one is unique, then one will necessarily perish: this is the price of individualism. So once there is only one leader without precedents and one God without competition, once there is no longer a place for multiplicity, death becomes a complete annihilation of the individual. As such it must be repressed and rejected" (ibid.). And indeed, after Akhenaten's death, polytheism was immediately restored and Akhenaten's legacy was brutally rejected. But one of Akhenaten's followers, an Egyptian man named Moses, probably an ambitious guy from an aristocratic family (and not, as the legend has it, a persecuted Hebrew baby saved by a compassionate Egyptian woman) sought to pursue monotheism further and looked for new disciples. The Hebrews, because of their inferior status, agreed to follow Moses, left Egypt and took upon them his new doctrine and his one-and-only God.

The identical traits between young Freud and his doctrine, and this literary twin of his are quite fascinating. The "first Moses" is described by Freud as an omnipotent, rational but also tyrannical leader who imposed harsh demands for religious exclusivity and loyalty and exhibited an uncompromising striving for an ultimate spiritual truth regarding his one almighty God. His doctrine did not leave room for magical thinking and satisfaction of primitive desires (both as believers who want to concretely worship and idolize their God and as anxious and deprived people who demanded compensation in their long, exhausting journey). Eventually, the Hebrews could not tolerate their demanding leader and assassinated Moses. Freud referred a few times in *Moses and Monotheism* to the similarity between the latter text to his earlier famous text *Totem and Taboo* (1913) and wrote that the Hebrews carried a repressed guilt over Moses' assassination, similar to the sons' guilt over the murder of the father figure in Totem and Taboo.

After introducing the first – Egyptian Moses, we are told by Freud of *a second Moses*, Moses the Midianite, who lived in Midian centuries later than the former one. This time we meet a very different and less omnipotent literary hero – as signified in the fact that he was stuttering. Quoting Meyer, Freud tells us: "Moses in Midian is no longer an Egyptian and grandson of Pharaoh, but a shepherd to whom Yahweh revealed himself." (Freud, 1939, p. 35). Years passed and a new Midianite leader whose name was also Moses was reminded of the first Moses' tradition that was passed between the generations, and sought a compromise between Jehovah – *a second God* of his time and the ancient God of Moses. His integrative offer was accepted by the local Israelites, thus creating also *a second group of Hebrew people* – a mixture of the offsprings of the first group who came from Egypt and the local residents. Freud recounts that this group of disciples believed in one God who was offered to them by this man of their time named Moses. According to the theory portrayed by Freud, the rehabilitation of Monotheistic belief in God offered a kind of reparation or at least a way for disavowal of the historical crime and guilt related to the assassination of the original Moses by his followers. Freud summarizes: "That in the course of long ages – between the Exodus from Egypt and the fixing of the text of the Bible under Ezra and Nechemiah some eight hundred years elapsed – the Yahweh religion had had its form changed back into conformity, or even perhaps into identity, with the original religion of Moses. And this is the essential outcome, the momentous substance, of the history of the Jewish religion." (Freud. 1939, p. 47).

The doubles are not only apparent in the historical reconstruction, but also manifested in the process of writing and publication of this text. As Freud himself testified, the text *Moses and Monotheism* itself was written in the course of five years, in which he published two parts in Vienna, and only when in London allowed himself to publish the third part, in which, according to his apologetic and heart rending testimony, a repetition could not be avoided: "Actually it has been written twice: for the first time a few years ago in Vienna, where I did not think it would be possible to publish it. I determined to give it up; but it tormented me like an unlaid ghost, and I found a way out by making two pieces of it independent and publishing them in our periodical *Imago*... Then, in March 1938, came the unexpected German invasion, which forced me to leave my home but also freed me from my anxiety lest my publication might conjure up a prohibition of psycho-analysis in a place where it was still tolerated... I did not succeed, however, in including the whole of this material in my second version; on the other hand I could not make up my mind to give up the earlier versions entirely. And so it has come about that I have adopted the expedient of attaching a whole piece of the first presentation to the second unchanged – which has brought with it the disadvantage of involving extensive repetition." (Ibid., pp. 103–104).

It is a great challenge to say something new about *Moses and Monotheism*, but at the same time, it is exactly this notion, of the challenge of claiming originality and singularity, "Mono-thesism" if you like, that Freud struggles with in this text. Moreover, repetition is not only unavoidable, it is at the core of this text. Interestingly enough, while so vividly and clearly portraying the history of the Hebrew people in two different phases, and with all the duplications I have presented above, Freud does not even once use the word "double" throughout the text. The literature researcher Eran Dorfman (2020) offers a thought-provoking interpretation of this, suggesting that "although Freud speaks of two figures of Moses and of two Jewish Gods, nowhere in his book does he mention the word 'double.' As such, the double is the repressed of the text, which nevertheless constitutes its secret motivation." (Dorfman, 2020, p.183).

I will now turn to read Freud's text regarding his transference relations to the different faces of Moses as Freud's literary twin.

Freud and His Literary Twins in *Moses and Monotheism* – a Psychoanalytic Perspective

Elsewhere (2020), I suggested that "reading literature often leads the reader to an encounter with 'twin heroes' who formulate for him what needs to be contained, worked through and articulated... The power of a 'transference twin' in literature stems from a combination of powerful feelings of identification and 'the distancing paradox'; that thinly veiled distance which enables the reader to be enriched by her literary twin. It is kind of 'non-identical twin' resembling a good interpretation in therapy echoing the patient's inner world but at the same time adding a further layer of some sort in terms of contents or in the way in which matters are worked through" (Roth, 2020, pp. 51–52).

There are several types of literary twins, some of which are found in *Moses and Monotheism*, each evoking a particular phantasy and unconscious process in the reader.

The first type of literary twins – the complementary twins – represents complementary traits characterized by both sides of a split. This type fits the following description by Freud: [Moses] "is often pictured as domineering, hot-tempered and even violent, yet he is also described as the mildest and most patient of men. These last qualities would evidently have fitted in badly with the Egyptian Moses, who had to deal with his people in such great and difficult matters; they may have belonged to the character of the other Moses, the Midianite. We are, I think, justified in separating the two figures and in assuming that the Egyptian Moses was never at Kadesh and had never heard the name of Yahweh, and that the Midianite Moses had never been in Egypt and knew nothing of Aten" (Freud, 1939, p. 41). The same split is relevant to the two Gods (perhaps in a contrary direction) – the rational God of Egypt and the Envious God of Midian.

In his Seminar VII Lacan (1959–1960), suggested that Freud identified with the Egyptian God and not with the God of the Midianites. "The rational God of the Egyptian Moses is the God Freud identifies with, the God of the love of logos, *amor intellectualis dei*, of Spinoza, of modern science that operates under the principle of 'the real rational and the rational real' (following Hegel)" (Benyamini, 2009 on Lacan, 1959–60).

I beg to differ on Lacan's interpretation, that in my view disregards the fact that literary reading offers the reader an opportunity to work through his own internal conflicts and pains through his identification with the various literary characters. Identification – the strongest magnet of literature – is experienced both consciously and unconsciously, and it is related to all the characters of a story, and not only to the idealized ones. One kind of hero – representing the reader's "ideal self" – is usually consciously (and always also unconsciously) identified by the reader. But no less an important part of working through is facilitated by the complementary literary twin – that of the twin villain – who holds for us the projected "bad" motivations and feelings that need metabolization and seek transformation. Freud needed these splitted aspects of the two Moses and two Gods, in order to work through different aspects of his personality, his historical choices and his changing motivations.

Moreover – the idealized hero is always also an intimidating figure, in introducing high standards and super-ego-like demands upon the reader. The first tyrannical Moses was indeed idealized in his love for truth and acknowledgment of sublimation and self-discipline, but he was also harsh and rigid as manifested in his demands, characteristic of an archaic and intimidating super-ego. The fact that he was then rejected by his disciples and finally murdered by them, might have offered the old reader Freud an opportunity to work through internal painful memories and fears. After the tragic fate of the rejected literary twin – Moses the first – his rehabilitated personification in the second literary twin – Moses the Midianite – offered Freud the reader an opportunity to work-through and reconcile himself with old wounds over various historical disappointments and betrayals (including by Otto Rank whose thesis Freud used in this text) and probably allowed some reparatory hope in the face of fears of future assassination by followers, readers and by the scientific community.

Totem and Taboo and *Moses and Monotheism* offer an alternative horizon to Freud's scientific prospect of the truth. In a paper written by Rachel Blass she writes: "The objective and detached stance that characterizes the classic view has the perception of reality, and reasoning about it, as the ultimate arbiters of truth. Doubt and error can be overcome through a scientific kind of study. In contrast, in the perspective on truth that emerges in Totem and Taboo, there are no such external measures to rely on. From this standpoint, Freud's propositions regarding early history cannot be tested, nor are they reasonable or necessary. As in his account of Moses, the measure of truth lies in the very conviction in their truth" (Blass, 2006, pp. 347–348). This idea supports our thesis that the story of the two Moses plays a role in Freud's internal processing of his own journey and of the horizon that awaited his "Torah" after his death. Similar to the two types of truth that Freud was finally maintaining, we can only imagine how the integrated and benign twins of second Moses and old Freud met many years after the much earlier encounter between the omnipotent twins of first Moses and young Freud, who took part in bloody battles in the name of their life-mission to spread their Torah and with it to change the history of human kind.

A second type of literary twins – the monstrous twins – shows similarity that is usually associated with perverted and murderous intentions and deeds. Edgar Allen Poe (1844) inserted a hint to the psychic activity of this kind of twinship involved in reading literature at the very end of his story "The purloined letter," where the hero, inspector Dupan, wrote a single sentence in the substituted letter which was left in the thief's apartment: "Such a baleful scheme, while not worthy of Atrée, is worthy of Thyeste" (Poe, 1844, p. 223). With these words the story by Poe ends, leaving it to the reader to discover that in Greek mythology Atrée et Thyeste were twin brothers, the sons of Pelops, who killed their half-brother, were exiled and subsequently fought each other for the throne of Mycenae. Following numerous unprecedented and violent intrigues, Thyeste murders his brother and becomes the unchallenged ruler of Mycenae. An important aspect that comes to life in such monstrous literary twins is the role of envy which plays a crucial part and might be the hidden drive behind the tyrannical and persecutory moralistic demands for exclusivity.

It is interesting for us to consider the need to murder in order to rule not only in terms of mythology, history, psychoanalysis, but also in terms of literature: The ruling of a writer is the death of his inspirations (Bloom, 1973), and the ruling of the reader is "The death of an author" (Barthes, 1967). In other words, the death of the author is both the cause of what the literary researcher Harrold Bloom (1973) named "The anxiety of influence" and a result of what Barth emphasized as the dominance of the reader as the main carrier of the text's meaning. The French philosopher Derrida (1980), who sees Poe's "Purloined letter" (1844) as a metaphor of literature, enables us to think of Freud the reader reflecting on the literary leaders Akhenaten and the first Moses as his monstrous twins, who 'murdered' their ancestors and then got murdered by their followers. In a sophisticated circulation – the ongoing envy and murderousness is what eventually promises immortality. As put by Dorfman: "How to face, then, posteriority? Freud, aware of the imminence of his disappearance, addresses his future readers and tells them that even if he is forgotten, one day someone will come across his writings and will know that 'there was someone in darker times who thought the same as you!' In other words, says Freud: you, the reader, are only my double. Perhaps you or your ancestors have killed me, but this only to guarantee my immortality: as every father, I am invincible. Even though I am hated in the present, even though I will soon die, I will find love and eternity through you: 'you! – hypocrite Reader!' – my double!' – my brother!" (Dorfman, 2020, p. 188).

A third type of literary twins – the Ideal twins – manifests heavenly goodness, often related to naïve innocence, as manifested in Moses the Midianite. Freud quotes Meyer writing: "The heroic character which the legend of his childhood presupposes is totally absent from the later Moses; he is only the man of God, a miracle-worker equipped by Yahweh with supernatural powers." (Freud, 1939, p. 36). In John Steiner's recent book (2020), he makes a wide and fascinating use of various literary sources to exemplify and clarify the psychic need of an illusion both as a defense as well as a basis for future development. Alongside "the dangerous gap between the real and the ideal" (ibid., p. 33), Steiner recognizes the developmental role of an ideal hero, to which, in the context of reading, I refer to as an ideal twin. Steiner suggests that we need "to differentiate between the ideal as a concrete belief on the one hand and as a symbol and measure of ideal goodness on the other. It also reveals the close parallel between the views of Milton and Klein both of whom believe that for healthy development an ideal object must initially be installed in the internal world" (Steiner, 2020, p. 36). We might consider two ideal objects in Freud's reconstruction of Moses' story. It seems that the early Moses was the young Freud's image of an ideal leader – strong, determined, persistent and devoted to an exalted mission. The second more integrated figure of Moses could serve as an ideal figure in the eyes of old Freud, who sees life with the wisdom of age, that Klein would see as a depressive position (1940). Unlike the total form of an ideal object characteristic of one side of the split in the paranoid-schizoid position (1946), this kind of an ideal literary twin helps the reader with **resignation in the face of reality** (Roth, 2020b) which I see as the encompassing mission of the depressive position. In Steiner's words: "If the narcissistic possession of the ideal can be relinquished and recognized to have been an illusion, the ideal object can be relinquished and mourned and in the process installed in the internal world as a symbol" (ibid., p. 37).

The combination of the **monstrous** and the **good twins** in one story represents not only the two sides of the split in the reader's psyche but also the vicissitudes between the paranoid-schizoid position and the depressive position in one's mind and life's fluctuations. In our case we could think of the unconscious working through that accompanies Freud's use of these various literary twins as a process in which the different faces of Moses transform along the timeline of the story which in Freud's analysis, takes the clear and concrete shape of First and Second. These enable Freud the reader to mobilize inner deadlocks according to the transformational journey of the characters – internal and external alike, offering him an opportunity to move from repetition to integration and even reparation.

The Art of Mourning

Elsewhere I suggested using Thomas Ogden's term of *the art of mourning* (Ogden, T., 2000) and point to a unique phenomenon that takes place in the course of reading which I termed the **reader's art of mourning**. "This phenomenon appears in all the psychic processes involved in the reading of literature and is a litmus test as to whether or not the reading becomes transformative. The transformative reading undermines the reader's long-established psychic equilibrium and transforms it *de novo*. It frees the reader of a variation of one kind or another of repetitive compulsion and psychic defences towards mobilization and the discovery of new creative pathways that will lead to reparation and renewal. This transformation involves the question as to whether the reader will use the reading in order to mourn the limitations of psychic and actual existence... Mourning of this kind is a necessary condition for negotiating one's way in life (internally and externally) despite the limitations of existence and even in light of those limitations" (Roth, 2020, pp. 303–304).

In the book by the existentialist philosopher Søren Kierkegaard, *Fear and Trembling – Dialectical Lyric* (1843) which in some intriguing ways parallels Freud's *Moses and Monotheism*, the narrator spends a lifetime of reading and re-reading the story of another Biblical hero – Abraham. Kierkegaard's narrator is trying to figure out Abreham's submission to God's demand that he shall sacrifice his own son. The narrator embarks on a years-long voyage of repeatedly reading just one text, a process derived from an intuitive belief that within that text he will ultimately resolve the moral riddle of Abraham – the textual hero of his life – and in doing so would be freed to mourn major missed opportunities in his life and to establish a renewed integration between his worldly and spiritual life.

I am using Kierkegaard's art of mourning enabled by reading Abraham's story, to shed light on Freud's art of mourning while reading Moses' story both through the similarities as well as through the differences between them.

Here are several striking similarities in the stories of Abraham and Moses: God is revealed to both heroes; Both heroes play a crucial part in the history of the Hebrew people; Both stories involve the threat of death of born sons; Circumcision (castration rituals) takes place in both stories; Both protagonists are invited to climb the mountain of God and both are requested to keep distant from their near fellows thus creating the very lonely existential and spiritual stand of a great leader (which is actually also the position of the greatest leader in the story – God, who testifies that "…man may not see Me and live" – Exodus, 33, 20); And both are requested to first Do and obey and then, if at all, Ask.

Kierkegaard struggles until he reaches the paradoxical notion, that Abraham's submission to God's demand to sacrifice his own son was not an act of masochism nor was it an act of moral heroism and also not that of a moral collapse. It was an act of deep resignation in the face of his limitations; knowing that he does not and cannot anticipate God's will and God's plan. This understanding frees Kierkegaard's narrator from his endless inner torture, and opens for him a space of reconciliation with his literary hero, and through him – with himself. He realizes that one cannot but put one's faith in his humble striving for a true and ethical attitude.

Unlike Abraham, Moses is chosen by God (and by Freud), not because he is a man of certainties and blind obedience but rather because he is struggling during every moment of his journey. The scope of this text does not allow me to investigate quite a few illuminating moments in the biblical story of Moses. However, inspired by Kierkegaard's discourse I do want to reflect on two paradigmatic (and cinematic) biblical pictures that are related to Moses apart from the exodus from Egypt. One is that of his furious breaking of the two stone Tablets of the Law on which the Ten Commandments were engraved (an act that was only briefly mentioned in Freud's *Moses and Monotheism* (Freud, 1939, p. 21). The second is old Moses on mount Nebo, gazing at the promised-land but not allowed to enter it. Freud did not interpret these pictures in his analysis of *Moses and Monotheism*, but since we do know that he was familiar with the biblical text, and since they play a crucial role in Freud's literary hero's story, we can allow ourselves to ask what they might represent.

The Breaking of the Stone Tablets – the Fate of a Leader

According to the biblical narrative, the first set of stone Tablets of the Law, inscribed by the finger of God (Exodus 31:18), was shattered by Moses when he was enraged by the sight of the Israelites worshipping a golden calf (Exodus 32:19). The second set of stone Tablets was later chiseled out by Moses according to God's directions (Exodus 34:1).

Let us think of this extraordinary moment. According to the Hebrew Bible, Moses was chosen by God to climb Mount Sinai and directly receive from him the two pieces of stone inscribed with the Ten Commandments. God is revealed to him, grants him this unprecedented honor, and Moses allows himself to break the stones because he is disappointed by the Israelites' regression to primitive beliefs and rituals. One can easily trace the resemblance between this overwhelming story and Freud's struggles and disappointments when bringing the psychoanalytic legacy to the scientific community at the beginning of his work, and in a sense throughout his whole endeavor as well. At this fragile moment, when the old, sick Freud leans on his desk to settle the text of *Moses and Monotheism,* the question of his legacy being kept and cherished was undoubtedly revived. Through his identification with Moses, Freud the reader was offered the opportunity to work through his own deep eagerness as a leader that his Torah will be accepted, and to mourn moments of great misery and rage – when, like Moses, instead of gratitude he was either betrayed by his followers or faced by indifference or blunt rejection by the scientific community. He can also mourn his own paranoid-schizoid moments of rivalry, resentments, and impulsive reactions. Through the revival of internal wounded objects which are always reflected in the literary story too, and through the reader's self-awareness of his own destructiveness in the face of his literary twin, the biblical story not only arouses guilt but also reveals the possibility of reparation, which is represented by the second Tablet of stones – recreating law and order and eventually handed to his people, allowing him a second chance after he 'lost it' in his temporary regression. The possibility and importance of reparation is signified by the content of the ten commandments as well, destined to be breached over and over again, yet one always has the internal option to rewrite them, re-member the pieces and repair what was formerly shattered (Roth, 2021).

Although at the time when *Moses and Monotheism* was published Freud was surrounded by loving family and friends and psychoanalysis was well-established, Moses' story also grants Freud an opportunity to work through and mourn his long lasting "sense of loneliness" (Klein, 1963) that is clarified in the biblical story to be an inherent position of a leader. Moses' face is so radiant after his encounter with the Lord, that "he put a veil over his face" (Exodus, 34:34). This radiance and veil that appear in a concrete form in the biblical story can also be read as a beautiful metaphor related to the time that is needed for the reader to get used to new insights and great influences. In this sense, we have here four levels of readers who need time to get used to the radiant message: Moses, who accepts the stones from God but is not allowed to see his face; The Israelites receiving the Ten Commandments from Moses but prove as immature and unready; Freud reading and writing the story of Moses several times and we reading Freud's interpretation of the story. We can also use this aspect of the radiance and the veil needed as a metaphor of a good interpretation, which should not dazzle or blind the patient who receives it but rather should be handed gently, perhaps somewhat veiled by its tremendous impact.

Mount Nebo and Psychoanalytic Nebo

In Deuteronomy 32:49–50, Moses receives another message from God, telling him the following: "Get thee up into this mountain of Abarim, unto mount Nebo, which is in the land of Moab, that is over against Jericho; and behold the land of Canaan, which I give unto the children of Israel for a possession; and die in the mount whither thou goest up, and be gathered unto thy people…"

Many interpretations were written on this heart-breaking ending of Moses, who, after an outstandingly challenging journey, was forbidden the privilege of entering the Promised Land of Israel with his people.

I suggest reflecting on this moment as a metaphor of the limitations of the psychoanalytic theory and practice in several senses:

First, Freud knew that although it is the target of the psychoanalytic investigation to unfold unconscious phantasies and motivations, it is clear by definition that one could never really "enter the unconscious land" – not of one's own nor of her analysands – but only see it from afar. "The narcissistic temptation to assert total control over the object of study through ideology or moral judgements is something of which historians, no less than clinicians, should be aware" (Rolnik, 2001, p. 147). The nearest we can come is to a Nebo mountain's vantage point – traced by the patient's free associations, dreams, and the like. Following this or said in another way, we can never really enter "the other." Freud knew that he could only reach that far into the other, even when that other tries as much as he can to allow him to invade his internal land.

Moreover, Moses' as well as Freud's grand legacies, or even Freud's small daily legacies in the shape of interpretations, could only be handed to others to carry into their world. But the wish to "escort them in," follow them, control, keep influencing etc. is blocked by at least two limitations:

a) They are handled by the other's unconscious, thus affected by various defenses - projected, denied and more – even when consciously "fully accepted."
b) Death keeps one apart from his followers, thus forces him to acknowledge the fact that toward the end of his life he is positioned on mount Nebo – and his followers are from now on out of reach and far from sight.

And lastly, our initial needs and wishes for complete unity and satisfaction with our desired object (including our transference object in analysis) is a phantasy of a Promised Land that we are bound to be expelled from and disappointed in. It is the land of partiality, separateness, and finitude that awaits us-all, and what psychoanalysis can help us with is to become reconciled to the human condition of Nebo-mountain in a depressive manner. And it is only from that vantage point, as Freud wrote in "On transience" (1916), that one can feel gratitude and appreciation toward the virtues that are growing in the land of reality.

Nevertheless, the story of Freud's literary twin, Moses, also offers a solution, or at least a consolation. As Franz Kafka wrote: "The expulsion from Paradise is in its main part eternal: so the expulsion from Paradise is indeed final, and life in the world inescapable, but the eternity of the process nevertheless makes it possible not only that we could remain in Paradise forever, but that in fact we are there forever, whether we know it here or not" (Kafka, 1931, p. 192).

And indeed, Moses does not fully accept his tragic fate of never reaching the promised-land. As the philosopher Micha Goodman wrote:

> Just before he died he delivered his life's greatest oration, full of ideas that were new, even revolutionary. He wrote down this parting address and it became a book, Deuteronomy, the fifth book of the Bible. It was Moses' final address that immortalized him… [in] Moses' final address… he expresses his dying wish not to remain on the eastern side of the Jordan but rather to be present among the people of Israel once they cross into the land. The measure of the success of his address lies in the enduring nature of his words. Again and again Moses enjoins the people to continue to invoke his address. They are commanded to write parts of it down on one of the stones on Mount Eyval when they enter the land. And when they appoint a king, it is incumbent upon that king to write down this speech and consult it throughout his reign. Furthermore, every seven years the nation is required to come together and listen to a public reading of Moses' final address. In the end, Moses did not enter the land, but it was his speech that entered the land in his stead
>
> (Goodman, 2022, pp. 2–3)

Freud's literary twin thus holds for both leaders (the hero and the reader) the leader's stick from its two ends (in both meanings): On the one hand and end – Moses acknowledges his limitations, declined from his omnipotent position, dying on Mount Nebo. On the other hand and end, he enters the land through his eternal legacy, landing Freud this literary consolation, in the shape of a horizon of a parallel "symbolic immortality" (Lifton, 1973), that of psychoanalysis that will live long after the death of its prophet.

Freud terminated his text by saying: "But exhaustive answers to such riddles cannot in fairness be either demanded or expected. A contribution, to be judged in view of the limitations which I mentioned at the start [p. 105], is all that I can offer" (Freud, 1939, p. 137). The story of his twin hero Moses on Nebo-mountain offered Freud-the-reader an opportunity to mourn not only his own limitations but also the limitations of his method, while at the same time to repair his wounded narcissism through the awareness of this state to be a universal human state that no one can escape. At the same time, the fact that Moses' image and legacy endured for centuries after his assassination by his followers, and again after his second, symbolic assassination, when left to die outside of the promised-land – also reflected what can and will remain from Freud's extraordinary life-work and endure long after he passed away. The force of universality as a remedy is one of literature's strongest reparatory powers. When Freud's literary twin is buried on Nebo-mountain, it might enable Freud to die with him with an internal reassurance that his image and legacy will be carried on and reach the Promised Land as many times as it will be explored by his readers, just like in this current reading of *Moses and Monotheism*.

Concluding Words

Like Perseus, who managed to overcome the Gorgon Medusa by viewing her reflection in his polished shield, so the readers of literature are enabled to approach their own story by viewing their reflection in their literary twins. Moreover,

> the reader uses literature as a way of transcending the circumstances of his existence. The reader ascends on the wings of the text to reach beyond his boundaries and then "returns" to himself the same and yet altered. The transcendence occurs in two central planes of the reader's existence; transcendence beyond the boundaries of self-identity and transcendence beyond the boundaries of the human body (and death).
>
> (Roth, 2020, p. 115)

This chapter suggested that Freud used Moses as his literary twin, and by viewing his reflection in the story of Moses which is full of grand dramas and radical moments of illusion and disillusion, Freud was able to reflect on his exceptional life's journey and transcend it all the way to the vantage points offered to him from the heights of Mount Sinai and Mount Nebo and all the other zeniths that Moses' story has lent him. I hope and believe that Freud's reading in *Moses* enabled him to gain new balance and integration between various aspects and manifestations of his internal and external worlds throughout his whole life journey. In a sense, reading and reflecting on the story of his twin hero Moses, which is also the history of the Jewish people, allowed the elderly Freud to write the final version of his own story, which is also the history of psychoanalysis.

Notes

1 "Portrait of an Old Man" is the name of a famous painting by Rembrandt (1645).
2 See for instance Freud's usage of E. T. A. Hoffman's "The Sandman" in "The Uncanny" paper (1919) and of Tasso's romantic epic "Gerusalemme Liberata" in "Beyond the Pleasure Principle" (1920).
3 It is hard to avoid the temptation to present one paragraph from *Totem and Taboo*, that brings forth Freud's interest in doubles in quite a remarkable way: "The two prohibitions which constitute its core – not to kill the totem and not to have sexual relations with a woman of the same totem – coincide in their content with the two crimes of Oedipus, who killed his father and married his mother, as well as with the two primal wishes of children, the insufficient repression or re-awakening of which forms the nucleus of perhaps every psychoneurosis." (Freud, 1913, p. 132).

References

Assmann, J. (1997). *Moses the Egyptian: The Memory of Egypt in Western Monotheism*. Cambridge, MA: Harvard University Press.

Barth, R. (1967). The Death of the Author. In: Lodge, David. (Ed.) *Modern Criticism and Theory – A Reader*. New York: Pearson Education Inc., pp. 145–150.

Benyamini, I. (2009). *Lacan's Discourse – The Revision of Psychoanalysis and Judeo-Christian Ethics*. Tel Aviv: Resling.

Bernstein, R. J. (1998). *Freud and the Legacy of Moses*. Cambridge: Cambridge University Press.

Blass, R. B. (2006). The role of tradition in concealing and grounding truth: two opposing Freudian legacies on truth and tradition. *Amer. Imago*, *63*(3), pp. 331–353.

Bloom, H. (1973). *The Anxiety of Influence – A Theory of Poetry*. New York: Oxford University Press.

Caruth, C. (1996). *Unclaimed Experience - Trauma, Narrative and History*. Baltimore: Johns Hopkins University Press.

Derrida J. (1980). *La Carte Postale: De Socrate a Freud et Au-Dela*. France: Flammarion.

Derrida, J. (1995). *Archive Fever: A Freudian Impression*, trans. Eric Prenowitz. Chicago: University of Chicago Press.

Dorfman, E. (2020). *Double Trouble – The Doppelgänger from Romanticism to Postmodernism*. London and New York: Routledge.

Freud, S. (1909). Family Romances. *S.E., Volume IX (1906–1908): Jensen's 'Gradiva' and* Other Works, London: Hogarth Press, pp. 235–242.

Freud, S. (1913). Totem and Taboo: Some Points of Agreement between the Mental Lives of Savages and Neurotics. *S.E., Volume XIII (1913–1914): Totem and Taboo and Other Works*, London: Hogarth Press, pp. vii–162.

Freud, S. (1914). The Moses of Michelangelo. *S.E, Volume XIII (1913–1914): Totem and Taboo and Other Works*, London: Hogarth Press, pp. 209–238.
Freud, S. (1916). *On Transience.* In: *S.E. Vol. XIV*, London: The Hogarth Press, pp. 303–307.
Freud, S. (1919). The Uncanny. In: *S.E. Vol. XVII*, London: The Hogarth Press, pp. 217–255.
Freud, S. (1920). Beyond the Pleasure Principle. In: *S.E. Vol. XVIII*, London: The Hogarth Press, pp. 1–64.
Freud, S. (1939). Moses and Monotheism. *S.E, Volume XXIII (1937–1939): Moses and Monotheism, An Outline of Psycho-Analysis and Other Works*, pp. 1–138.
Goodman, M. (2022). *Moses' Final Address*. Jerusalem: Koren.
Kafka, F. (1931[2012]). *A Hunger Artist and Other Stories.* Oxford: Oxford University Press.
Kierkegaard, S. (1843[2003]). *Fear and Trembling*. London: Penguin.
Kierkegaard, S. (1844[1985]). *Philosophical Fragments*. Trs. and Eds: H. V. Hong and E. Hong. Princeton: Princeton University Press.
Klein, M. (1940). Mourning and Its Relation to Manic-Depressive States. In: *Love, Guilt and Reparation and other works 1921–1945.* London: Vintage, pp. 344–369.
Klein, M. (1946). Notes on Some Schizoid Mechanisms. In: *Envy and Gratitude and Other Works 1946–1963.* London:Vintage, pp. 25–42.
Klein, M. (1963). On the Sense of Loneliness. In: *Envy and Gratitude and Other Works 1946–1963.* London: Vintage, pp. 300–313.
Lacan, J. (1959-60). The Ethics of Psychoanalysis. (Ed.) J. A. Miller*: Écrits: A Selection – Book VII.* New York and London: W.W. Norton and Company.
Lifton, R. J. (1973). The Sense of Immortality: On Death and the Continuity of Life. *Am. J. Psychoanal.*, 33(1), pp. 3–15.
Ogden, T.H. (2000). Borges and the Art of Mourning. *Psychoanal. Dial.*, *10*(1), pp. 65–88.
Poe, E. A. (1844[2011]). The Purloined Letter. In: *The Complete Works of Edgar Allan Poe*. Orange Sky Project – Kindle Edition.
Rolnik, E. J. (2001). Between Memory and Desire: From History to Psychoanalysis and Back. *Psychoanal. Hist.*, *3*(2), pp. 129–151.
Roth, M. (2020). *A Psychoanalytic Perspective on Reading Literature – Reading the Reader*. London and New York: Routledge.
Roth, M. (2020b). The Death Drive Is Alive and Kicking. *Sihot – Israeli J. of Psychotherapy*, *35*-I, pp. 24–30.
Roth, M. (2021). Every Day We Must Rewrite the Tablets of the Law. Israel: *HaAretz Newspaper*, May 27, 2021.
Said, E. W. (2003). *Freud and the Non- European.* London: Verso.
Steiner, J. (2020). *Illusion, Disillusion, and Irony in Psychoanalysis*. London and New York: Routledge.
Yerushalmi, Y. H. (1991). *Freud's Moses: Judaism Terminable and Interminable.* New Haven, CT: Yale University Press.

Editor's Introduction to Chapter 5

Lawrence J. Brown

In this chapter, Sara Collins examines the essential significance that truth, especially *historical truth*, plays in *Moses and Monotheism*. She notes that the act of remembering, regardless of the age and origin of that which is remembered, "takes place in the service of the here and now." In this last book of Freud's, we see him reaching back to some of his earlier concepts and applying these in new and fresh ways: he borrows from the earlier notion of latency in which the erotic drives of the oedipal stage were driven into repression and applies this model of individual psychological development to account for an historical event disappearing from *collective* memory, such as the murder of Moses. Similarly, Freud (1921) applied his earlier writings on the nature of group psychology to explain the complex relationship – sometimes idealized and not infrequently embittered – between the members of a group and its leader. Collins also highlights the importance of Freud's paper, "Constructions in analysis" (1937), written contemporaneously with the last chapter of *Moses and Monotheism*, as a "paradigm for reconstructing early childhood memories" just as an archaeologist may strive to recreate a long-forgotten society from shards of pottery.

Collins presents an interesting clinical vignette of a 12-year-old boy with a fetish to illustrate the potential value of reconstructions in analytic practice, but cautions us that "analytic constructions of early infantile memories cannot be taken as ultimate truths. They are only probabilities." Furthermore, she asserts that analytic constructions are impermanent and "they are likely to depend on the context of the transference in the analytic field." Reconstructions of the patient's past always take place in the present; therefore, Collins argues, that the ongoing transference situation in treatment will affect the patient's recollections of his/her past. She also asserts that "although it [historical past] is a story about the past, it is also a representation of a present experience in the analysis, which, in turn, seeks to internally alter and heal recovered aspects of past."

DOI: 10.4324/9781003272045-10

5 Memory and Historical Truth in *Moses and Monotheism*

The Contemporary Significance of "Historical Truth"

Sara Collins

Preamble

The act of remembering is an act in a present moment. The content of what is remembered is of something that is not of the present moment, but of moments past. Whether it is of a recent time or long ago, it is deemed to be "the past" or "history." While the subject matter of what is remembered is considered to be not of our current experience, the act of recollection takes place in the service of the here and now. We trust what is in front of us which we witness, participate in emotionally, and believe it to be true. It is, at the very least, authentic. However, what it is we designate as "past" and "history" becomes less reliable in its truthfulness. The time lapse between the ascribed time of occurrence and the moment of recall opens up questions of reliability. It is in that gap that profound and significant dialectics exist on the attribution of historical truth.

Freud was engaged with the relationship between the essential elements of memory, truth, and historical truth in his writings, and this investigation continues. Of particular relevance is the question of what kind of truth is being investigated and constructed in the analytic dialogue; and how does the analyst go about it. Therefore, it is of interest to explore Freud's interrogation of notions of memory and historical truth in *Moses and Monotheism*. These inter-related concepts were a conundrum he was occupied with throughout his working life.

It is curious why Freud chose *Moses and Monotheism* as a subject for examination, which seemingly has little to do with the "talking cure" which takes place in the privacy of the consulting room. As well, he turned to wide ranging subjects from history, culture, anthropology, archaeology, and literature, and across a large time span of knowledge.

"My construction starts out from a statement of Darwin's [1871, 2, 362 f.] and takes in a hypothesis of Atkinson's [1903, 220 f.]" (Freud, 1939, p. 31).

This might be part of his relentless testing of the project of psychoanalysis against wider scientific subjects, outside the clinical practice of psychoanalysis, so as to offer further affirmation and validity to his

DOI: 10.4324/9781003272045-11

thinking on a universal model of the mind. In face of much opposition to his ideas at the time, Freud was at once testing the reach of psychoanalysis, and demonstrating its increasing domain of applicability to all aspects of human experience. During his last days, Freud devoted his time to work on *Moses and Monotheism*, which he called 'My Moses,' on what was to be his death bed. It is believed that his choice of Moses and the related inquiry into the origins of the Jewish faith was partly in response to the rise of Nazism in Europe during his time. It was also a way of dealing with the painful cancer of the jaw which beleaguered him for many years, and became intolerable at the end. Arguably, this was an identification with the figure Moses, whose capacity to communicate was also hampered by a speech impediment.

In this book Freud tested his theory of infantile sexuality and human development through the well-known historical narrative of the formation of the Jewish nation. This he did by drawing an analogy between the history of Jews and the psychoanalytic principles of conflict, repression, and the gap of latency in human development. He maintained that Moses had been killed by the Israelites, the knowledge of which was then repressed by the group. Having been forgotten, it had entered a long period of being unavailable to memory. Until that is many generations later, when the memory had begun to surface, in a way analogous to the re-emergence of conflicts during adolescence. The project of *Moses and Monotheism* was a subject of great relevance to his own relationship with his Jewishness and to his intellectual confrontation with spiritual belief, and its function in the human mind. In this text he sought to apply the ideas of psychoanalysis to group psychology, expanding the scope of psychoanalysis beyond that of the individual psyche to multifaceted aspects of social, religious, and cultural life.

Introduction

The aim of this chapter is not to enter into a dialogue with the contents of the book and its assertions. Rather, the focus will be the nature of the *methodology* Freud uses in his understanding of the narration of the historical figure Moses, as essentially a story of constructed memory and historical truth. It examines how, and by use of which scholarly sources Freud pieces together his thesis on the man Moses and the onset of the Jewish religion. Primarily, it is an application of psychoanalytic concepts to the important functions of memory. Freud does this by applying the "construction" model, a paradigm for reconstructing early childhood memories, as set out in "Constructions in analysis" (Freud, 1938).

Freud recounts his story of *Moses and Monotheism* by using ethnological, historical, and Egyptology scholars. As well, he does that by applying his own earlier writing on *Totem and Taboo* (1912–1913), and the later writing on reconstruction. The main contention of the book is that the Mosaic religion was based on an amalgamation of two great figures known as Moses, separated by a few generations, the first Moses having been murdered by his people. The explanations given for these events are based on the, by then, established psychoanalytic principles of infantile trauma, repression, latency, and the return of the repressed. All of which are fully explicated in 'Constructions in psychoanalysis' (ibid.). It is perhaps not a co-incidence that Freud designates the archaeologist as his model investigator of human beginnings, since he was steeped in antiquity and Egyptology. Being an antiquities enthusiast, Freud famously collected ancient artefacts, making regular trips to an antiques' dealer in Vienna. He lived in a period of great interest in all things Egyptian, following the discoveries along the Nile, greatly acclaimed by the scientific community.

The first two essays of *Moses and Monotheism* were originally published in 1937 [in *Imago* 23 (1), 5–13 and (4), 387–419.] At the end of the same year, in December 1937, Freud published his paper 'Constructions in Analysis.' It was to be one of his last works. Both essays deal with the healing power of recovered memory in psychoanalysis. This is done by unearthing forgotten events and establishing the historical truth of childhood memories through imaginative reconstruction on part of the analyst. At the same time there are indications, and seeds of thoughts in Freud's late writings; questions and doubts Freud was wrestling with on the very nature of truth, historical truth, and their relation to what he called material truth. That is, the extent to which the uncovered memories the analyst is dealing with are objective real truths or subjectively constructed truths. The editorial note to 'Constructions in analysis' states:

> The paper ends with a discussion of a question in which Freud was much interested at this period – the distinction between what he described as 'historical' and 'material' truth.
>
> (Standard Edition, p. 256)

Freud did not live to elaborate on these questions. However, psychoanalysts have continued to explore and debate these seminal concepts of truth, memory, and historical truth. This chapter explores significant implications of these debates for contemporary psychoanalytic theory and practice.

Present day analytic thinking has advanced these inquiries, giving them a current perspective as well as providing a springboard for further discussions and understanding the nature of memory. That is, how remembering functions in the context of present moments within the analytic relationship. Of particular interest are current dialogues on the analytic third and the analytic field. Questions like: How does historical memory function in the here and now of the intersubjective field? What is the meaning of "historical truth" when memories converge within the dyad of the analytic encounter, when analyst and patient share similar childhood memories, though in different contexts? Do patients unconsciously trigger personal memories in the analyst and if so, by which mechanism? Or is it the other way round? And whose "truth" is it anyway?

The 'Yawning Gap' in History: Latency and Its Relation to Memory

A striking assertion in *Moses and Monotheism* is that there were two people leading the Israelites in ancient times named Moses, who became amalgamated into one. The other notable claim is that Moses was an Egyptian and not a Jew, thus asserting that the introduction of Monotheism predates the Israelites. Monotheism existed in ancient Egypt as the religion of Aten, at the period it was a world empire. This religion consisted of worshipping the sun as the omnipotent source of all life giving, representing an absolute and singular power. It was a monotheistic religion of a high intellectual level, shunning excess mysticism and superstitions, and promoting developed ethical values of everyday life. This original monotheistic religion of Aten eventually came to grief, but its traditions continued to be adhered to in a minority of people to which Moses belonged, and he introduced it to the Jews. The Egyptian Moses was the first one historically. Then there was a second Moses who became a leader of the Israelites after a long gap of several hundred years. This second one was a Midianite, a polytheistic people, who worshipped the god Yahweh as one of their numerous gods at the time. While Aten was an enlightened sun god, Yahweh was harsh and vengeful. According to Freud, the second, Midianite Moses had never been to Egypt, and knew nothing of the first Mosaic religion that stemmed from Aten. But the glorious mantle of Monotheism, initially espoused by the Egyptian Moses, descended on the Midianite, second Moses. Thus, Freud (1939) states, the Biblical story of Moses was a narration of history with not a little impartiality. And this he relates to the general malleability of early memories:

> Long-past ages have a great and often puzzling attraction for men's imagination. Whenever they are dissatisfied with their present surroundings… they turn back to the past and hope that they will now be able to prove the truth.... They are probably still under the spell of their childhood, which is presented to them by their not impartial memory as a time of uninterrupted bliss.
>
> (p. 71)

There was a murder involved in the story. The original Moses had been killed by the people he led, in an act of primitive parricide, thus comparing the Israelites at the time to ancient tribes of primordial times. Their customary habit it had been to eliminate the father, conceived as a rival for the possession of the females in the group (See "Totem and Taboo,"

1912–1913). This would have been the only way for sons to achieve procreation, an instinctual demand that took precedence over inhibitions of morality. No surprise then, that the sordid event was forgotten. This provided for Freud a lively example of the work of "repression," in a past historical time, and of how guilt had played its part in it.

Only a few of the first Moses followers, the Levites, carried on his traditions, perhaps in secret. Until, that is, it was time, after a very long gap for the memory of the original Moses to resurface in the people's consciousness; inevitably so, it seemed, according to Freud's principle of the 'return of the repressed.' Freud focused on this lapse of time in Jewish history, as equivalent to latency in human development. Its particular revelatory aspect, however, was that far from implying this was a phase of no psychic activity, it was a time when the repressed memory continued to exist in the unconscious, and so to speak "ferment trouble" in there. Then, following this principle of "symptom formation," a compromise was established between the opposing needs of repression and expression. In the story of Moses this appeared in the form of a new figure Moses on whom the mantle of Monotheism descended, through being amalgamated in the people's minds with the earlier Moses. The two Mosaic leaders were thus welded into one, and an uninterrupted narrative of the formation the Jewish people was created. However, for this to have happened, a murder was covered up, hidden within the fabric of the large intricate canvas of history.

As a rule, Freud in his enquiries was especially interested in gaps, interruptions, and the spaces between. He continually explored the meaning of what was missing, what was *not* said. Alongside dreams, the phenomena of gaps, hesitations, and forgetting he maintained that all were all points of entry to the unconscious. For example, he famously discovered the concept of resistance when his patients fell silent in the middle of a stream of free associations (Psychopathology, 1901b). Jokes too, that related to gaps and absences were explored for their unconscious meaning (*Five Lectures on Psychoanalysis*, 1910a).

In *Moses and Monotheism* (1939) Freud explored the vagaries of collective memory, through examining the outcome of the time lapse between the lives of the two mosaic leaders. For this he coined the metaphorical term of 'the yawning gap' (pp. 1–138); a significant disparity that demanded explanation. He advanced the psychoanalytic explanation of compromise between opposing psychic forces. That is, between the need for repressing the guilt associated with a dishonorable murder, and the growing need, increasing over time, for the re-awakening of the old memory associated with it. It was of the Egyptian Moses and his invaluable monotheistic principles, while at the same time keeping the murder under wraps. In this, the parallel is to the compromises involved in symptom formation, which are at once a psychic solution for keeping the repression, while providing some expression of it, in the form of a mnemic symbol of the original traumatic event.

> The Jewish people had abandoned the Aten religion brought to them by Moses… All the tendentious efforts of later times failed to disguise this shameful fact. But the Mosaic religion had not vanished without leaving a trace; some sort of memory of it had kept alive – a possibly obscured and distorted tradition… which gradually acquired more and more power over people's minds and which in the end succeeded… in re-awakening into life the religion of Moses that had been introduced and then abandoned long centuries before.
>
> (ibid., pp. 69–70)

In the Moses historical narrative, Freud emphasizes a similarity between this tribal story and the life of the individual. He draws a direct analogy with children's mental life, that follows the same developmental process of repression and latency, at the end of which sexual conflicts reappear in new forms. Like the Moses account, the emergence of sexual maturity too requires a compromise with earlier infantile anxieties related to aggression. What stands out from this comparison between a historical gap and the individual latency period, is the emphasis on the role of memory, which is juxtaposed with repression and its associated outcome.

A Freudian notion, distinguished from memory, though related to it, is that of acting out. Thus, Freud sees the subsequent adoption of the monotheistic idea, many years after the killing of Moses, as a form of action in place of remembrance. Or, put another way, *acting is a (compromised) form of remembering*. In the context of *Moses and Monotheism*, the act of adopting Monotheism by the Jews, long after their ancestors had murdered its exponent Moses, was an expression of the "return of the repressed" through action, circumventing a direct memory. However, that reawakening of a long forgotten past, being a compromise between repression and its return, has consequences, in the form of significant biases and fabrications. Rather like symptoms which are "mnemic symbols" of a forgotten past trauma, the returned memory does not reappear in its original form. It is symbolically represented and its "historical truth" is subjected to distortions. Freud maintains that those who had come from Egypt, had subsequently written their own history, and incorporated in it psychic concessions to their unconscious guilt.

> All the phenomena of the formation of symptoms may justly be described as the 'return of the repressed.' Their distinguishing characteristic, however, is the far-reaching distortion to which the returning material has been subjected as compared with the original.
>
> pp. 126–127

Monotheism and Its Constructions: The Archaeological Model

"The killing of Moses by his Jewish people… thus becomes an indispensable part of our construction, an important link between the forgotten event of primaeval times and its later emergence in the form of the monotheist religions" (p. 89).

Freud established the vital link between psychopathology, forgetting, and the healing power of enabled recollection. Remembering and reconstructing childhood traumatic events, in and of itself, can provides the essential elements for subsequent restoration and recovery. "Recovery," in this context, has the double meaning of finding and healing.

In "Constructions in Analysis" (1938) Freud presents an analogy between the work of the psychoanalyst and that of the archaeologist. Regarding the question of uncovering an individual's "historical 'truths,'" he compares human memory to layers of earth, where the oldest remnants of ancient civilizations would lie deepest; the various levels relating to stages of historical times. For example, a shard of a Grecian vase would be buried at a deeper level than that of a Roman and so on. The role of the psychoanalyst is similar to that of the archaeologist. Both are in search of evidence for what was once there. The task is like a fact-finding mission for something as concrete and real as an ancient coin.

"What we are in search of is a picture of the patient's forgotten years that shall be alike trustworthy and in all essential respects complete" (p. 258).

This, according to Freud, is indispensable for the analytic work of "construction," by which he means presenting to his patients the full story of an important childhood experience, put together by the analyst, aided by the patient's own uncovered memories. This way, Freud maintains, it is possible to explain to patients their symptoms, to offer insight, and to make them feel understood, which ultimately leads to relief from suffering.

The earliest forgotten event, the one closer to beginning of life, would be the most deeply repressed, representing a more primitive stage of development, when the capacity for representation is yet to be securely developed and is more vulnerable to disruption. And so, it lies at the furthest reaches of the unconscious, is more likely to be fragmented, and the task of reconstruction is more complex. It also presents the greatest resistance. In terms of the archaeologic metaphor, the more primitive the infantile pathogenic event, the more difficult to reach it would be, and the harder to unearth and recover its original shape.

The mission of historical recovery in an archaeological dig is twofold. The first aim is the finding of evidence, which comes in the form of material proof, such as shards of pots, jewelry, bones, and so on. Then follows the task of constructing a story of the lives of the people at that time. This is done by the painstaking work of piecing together, say, fragments of a vase, and reconstructing it to its previous shape. There will, inevitably, be pieces missing, which will be recreated by way of conjecture. A vase, for example, will be imaginatively restored by following shapes and contours of other similarly found items. There will be an assumption, an imagining of what the rest of the story would be like, so that a comprehensive narrative of the time would be assembled, which is when the archaeologist's task is completed.

Some Limitations of the Archaeological Model

The metaphorically rich evocations of the archaeological model have remained in the foreground of discussions on constructions in psychoanalysis, and have drawn equally strong reservations by later psychoanalytic writings. However, already Freud (1938) drew a distinction in his comparison between psychoanalytic construction and the archaeological model, by stating that the two disciplines part company at the moment of discovery. He held that whereas getting the find would be the aim for the archaeologist, who does not need to interact with objects in order to confirm his hypotheses, for the psychoanalyst this is only the beginning of analytic work. It starts by putting the reconstruction to the patient, and waiting for the patient's *affective* response to it. According to Freud, it is necessary to recover not only the "factual" memory (this or that event happened), but crucially, the emotional memory, which could not have been experienced at the time.

With too great an emphasis on the analogy between the scientist with his/her tools at an archaeological dig, a view was created of the neutral, distant, and affectless analyst, famously coined as "the blank screen." Whereas, I maintain, Freud repeatedly emphasized the centrality of affect in the psychoanalytic encounter. This from early writings, for example in "Five lectures on psychoanalysis" (1910), where he stressed that the recovery of repressed memory cannot achieve its healing effect and change in symptoms, unless it is accompanied by the appropriate amount of affect; its repression being the primal cause of the symptoms in the first place. Remembering is accompanied by re-experiencing what had been forgotten, according to Freud. Later, as will be discussed below, this was further developed into an understanding that remembering is not only about re-experiencing, but also about the capacity to experience for the first time emotions that could not find representation (Bion, 1956, 1959, 1962). This was thought to be due to conflicts, according to Freud. Or, as Winnicott (1974), and Bion held, due to insufficient environmental response, preoccupation/reverie and lack of maternal containment. In short, memory, affective representation, and constructions are closely interwoven.

The Freudian concept of memory, which functions as "recollection" and "recovery" of long forgotten past events, including its attendant affects, has a robust fit with *Moses and Monotheism*. But Freud's main thesis in this book expands on his earlier notions of memory, in the sense that it also considers *changes* to the memory that occur over the course of time. In the process of re-emergence of the original Moses and his invaluable legacy of

Monotheism, the recall of the murderous event of killing him, in a primal act of parricide, had been transformed and remodeled.

Another aspect limiting the epistemic value of the archaeological model is its reliance on insufficient evidence. The discovered elements are likely only small fragments of a whole.

> … .it must be borne in mind that the excavator is dealing with destroyed objects… No amount of effort can result in their discovery and lead to their being united with the surviving remains. The one and only course open is that of reconstruction, which for this reason can often reach *only a certain degree of probability*.
>
> (Freud, 1938, p. 260, italics added)

And: "Constructions are a 'probable historical truth'" (ibid., p. 291).

This is not unlike Elliot's (1935) statement that the past is always only "a perpetual possibility" (p. 177).

In summary, analytic constructions of early infantile memories cannot be taken as ultimate truths. They are only probabilities. As well as lacking certainty they also lack permanence. In other words, they are temporary. My contention is that they are likely to fluctuate and change along the progression of the analytic process. Remembrances can mutate and be altered along the development of relationships with patients. I would also maintain that they are likely to depend on the context of the transference in the analytic field. In other words, on the time and phase a specific memory recovery takes place.

A Clinical Example

Fabian, of mixed-race heritage and from an African country, felt compelled to put on women's stockings and shoes since the age of 12. It became a lifelong secretive fetish, which always filled him with excitement and anxiety. He came to treatment after he had been seen by a work colleague dressed as a woman. This precipitated a crisis in his life. Up to that point, he had led a "double life," living both as a man and a woman, but the two modes of living were strictly separated.

It seemed he had an unconscious wish to end the exhausting split in his life, and find a way of accommodating being in both male and female clothing, with its significant psychic meanings and attendant identifications. Toward the end of the analysis, he felt able to exert fewer controls over the split in his external gender appearance, and in how he dressed. He allowed himself to be with the same people, sometimes appearing as a male and at others as a female, whose acceptance of his alternating looks reassured him, and he settled on describing himself as "sexually nonbinary" and as "a gender enhanced male."

At the beginning of treatment, I asked Fabian to tell me about the first memory he had of putting on his mother's clothes as a child. Then, three years into the treatment Fabian was beginning to construct his own life history and again talked about the onset of his fetish. These two historical accounts were remarkably different in context, though both were told with equal conviction in their historical truth. The patient was not aware of the difference between the two accounts of onset.

The First Time

He was walking in the street, age 12, when he happened to look through an open window. He saw a pair of high heeled shoes lying on the floor and instantly felt attracted to them. This, he said, was how he developed a compulsion to look at women's legs and shoes wherever he was. And it was then that he started wearing his mother's shoes.

The Second Time

Again, he was 12, but this time his attraction to shoes started when he was at home. He said he saw a magazine article lying on the kitchen table about the harmful effects of high-heeled shoes on women's legs and backs. He felt concern for his mother, who wore stiletto shoes, and went to the bedroom to look at her shoes and try them on. He immediately felt an exquisite pleasurable sensation and found himself compelled to step into them whenever he had the opportunity to do so.

The Contemporary Transferential Context

In understanding the difference between the two versions the patient reported, the analyst examined the transference at each of the analytic periods, in terms of the quality of the patient's connection with his objects and with the analyst when each of the historical versions was told.

In the first account of onset, the patient was in the street, looking into a room of an anonymous person who was not there. At this initial stage, the patient's relationship with the analyst was very distant. He was talking in a pressurized manner, as though seeking relief from his troubled mind by emptying it, but not having room to take in the analyst's presence. The analyst was treated as a part-object – a pair of ears without a personality of her own. When talking about his childhood at the early stage, the patient stated that his mother was of no great significance for him, and had no presence in his life. The family was dominated by an exacting sadistic father, who was a successful litigations solicitor. He demanded high achievement from his son, and controlled the family by scornful and cutting witticisms; on several occasions he humiliated his son in public.

The analyst talked to Fabian about his dread, when he first saw her, of a denigrating and cutting authority. This was understood as reflecting his fantasy of being cut to size by someone with authority. He revealed that he had expected the analyst to advise him to undergo a sex change operation which would involve removing his penis, and that he would have to follow it. He could not imagine any other moderating view other than that. At that time, he could not yet experience me in the transference as a mitigating maternal presence. To protect himself from the fantasied threat of castration, he kept the analyst at a distance, as the blank, unidentified person, similar to the context of the historical beginning of his symptoms.

Before the second account of onset the patient talked at some length about his mother, and told the analyst that she had died some year before. He was surprised, he said, at having omitted her from his memory so completely, and for the first time he allowed himself to experience grief and sadness at her loss. At this stage the patient began to feel more at ease when he came into the room, and to allow a dialogue and interchange with his analyst, as well as recognizing feelings of sadness and loss before analytic breaks. The shift in the scenes of the two accounts of onset is significant, as it moves from an anonymous external place to an internal, familiar location. It is significant that the second version contains an expression of concern for his objects, a worry about his mother's back. This, unlike the dismissive attitude to the mother at the beginning. Both accounts mirrored stages in the transference, and their quality of relatedness to the analyst.

I believe this shows that a reconstruction of the past, which takes place in the present, can be greatly affected by the contemporaneity of telling. That is, the historical past is seen through a prism of the actual moment of communicating. Like a prism, which alters and refracts the light coming into it, so that the light coming out of it is changed, so can the transference alter aspects of memory. It affects the construction of historical truth, so as to account for, and express, essential affects prevailing in the analytic field during the experience of telling (Spence, 1982). Therefore, although it is a story about the past, it is also a representation of a present experience in the analysis, which, in turn, seeks to internally alter and heal recovered aspects of past.

Further Reservation of the Archaeological Model: Bion

At the 1957 International Congress Bion (1959) critiqued Freud's archaeological model used in *Moses and Monotheism*:

> I suggested that Freud's analogy of an archaeological investigation with a psycho-analysis was helpful if it were considered that we were exposing evidence not so much of a primitive civilization as of a primitive disaster… in the analysis we are confronted not so much with a static situation that permits leisurely study, but with a catastrophe that

remains at one and the same moment actively vital and yet incapable of resolution into quiescence.

The archaeological model centered on what is found *after* the destruction of a civilization. Its resultant fragmentation having settled into the depth of earth, the scientist wants to know how it can be re-constructed. Bion's (1959) attention focused on the actual dynamics of disintegration in the human psyche and its consequences, as it were in real time. He explained it as a primitive defense against devastating pain and trauma that could not have psychic representation, therefore not experienced [this, perhaps not surprising given his experiences of the desolations of WWI]. His observations of psychotic patients attested to the fact that they appeared not to dream, or at least not to know about their dreaming, since the raw material of their dreams was "so minutely fragmented that they are devoid of any visual component" (ibid., p. 310).

Bion saw mental devastation as being a dynamic ongoing process that occurs each time the patient attempts to think. Unlike a static state post destruction, for example, in Pompei, which once destroyed people and objects remained in fixed petrification, primitive psychic attacks are active and constant. As any attempt at thinking is felt dangerous, it is immediately attacked, and the patient has no memory nor dreams. The result is a continuous lack of curiosity and an incapacity to learn. Bion investigated the disruption of dreaming as an assault on a basic function of the work of the unconscious. In other words, "dreaming" is a psychic achievement which exists in normal development, and the incapacity to dream results from primitive disturbances in patients too psychically damaged to muster it. This is because they developed a hatred of emotions, and Bion (1959) equates the hatred of emotion with the hatred of life itself. This sorrow state comes about due to catastrophic failure in containment, when the infant is confronted with an inaccessible object, who is incapable of accepting projections, essential for reducing psychic toxicity.

"The internal object which in its origin was an external breast that refused to introject, harbour, and so modify the baneful force of emotion, is felt, paradoxically, to intensify, relative to the strength of the ego, the emotions against which it initiates the attacks" (pp. 314–315).

The difference between Freud and Bion hinges on aspects of representation. According to Levine (2021), Freud sees archaeological remains as representing a psychic event that had been repressed, but has remained in the unconscious in some retrievable form, which can be recovered through memory. Bion, however, would see the traumatic event as having caused fragmentation beyond recognition, with the result that the capacity for visual representation is fractured beyond recovery by ordinary means of "remembering."

Nevertheless, the important function of dream recollection emphasized by Bion can be viewed as aligned with Freud's focus on the recovery of early pathogenic events, in the sense that both relate to early childhood, and involve the primary work of the unconscious in relation to infantile events. The difference however is that for Freud recollection is clearly linked with some form of re-instatement, of something already experienced, and then repressed, as the term "return" in "return in the repressed" would indicate. For Bion, on the other hand, dreaming gives representation to emotional experience through the process of alpha function, that is a primary psychic process that generates meaning in the form of a thought to an experience for the very first time.

The classical analytic task in the consulting room is to enable the retrieval of unconscious elements of early experiences, and to re-construct them into a historical narrative. For the Bionian psychotic state of mind, in which representation had been shattered into unrecognizable shapes, a fundamental function of linking is missing. These patients are unable to remember; they can only enact.

Therefore, the analytic task would be markedly different, following Bion and further developments in understanding of intersubjectivity. The analyst, in a state of reverie, and through the understanding of the countertransference, uses his/her own psyche so to speak, in the service of the patient. The analyst, then, is a kind of "proxy unconscious," to be temporarily utilized in place of the patient's impoverished unconscious. This way, through unconscious communications within the analytic dyad, the analyst offers a channel for potential transformation. Developments in understanding the intersubjective field uniquely afford new understanding of different pathways (Brown, 2019; Birksted-Breen, 2019; Ogden, 2017) to the analyst's unconscious from the patient, for what had been consistently deconstructed and unrepresented. And in this way the analytic process assists the patient's recovery. Therefore, following Bionian thinking with its attendant advances in theory of practice, psychoanalysts moved away from the "blank screen," the emotionless and the so-called neutral analyst, often associated with earlier periods of psychoanalysis (Collins, 2015).

Additionally, the emphasis shifted from narration of historical truth in neurotic presentations, which are more likely to be available for recall, to the more disturbed cases early trauma, in which representation and memory are severely disrupted.

Historization of Trauma

Freud conception of trauma is as an event at which the psyche is overwhelmed by intrusive negative stimulation, which it is unable to process, so as to restore stability. In *Moses and Monotheism*, he illustrated these ideas by expounding on the trauma of the Israelites who had murdered Moses, and on the consequent guilt suffered, that had to be repressed and forgotten. Elsewhere, Freud (1920) elaborated on the essential riddle of trauma, which is its repetition; the compulsive unconscious need to replicate unwanted negative experiences. This contrasts with the need for equilibrium (nirvana) in the psychic system. The answer, Freud maintained, lay in an attempt at integration, a hope that next time, if the stimulus was to be presented in a smaller, less toxic portion so to speak, the individual might not be overwhelmed, the experience integrated by the ego and coped with. Thus, the reawakening of the memory of the original Moses, created a need felt by the Israelites to integrate his legacy and invaluable contribution of Monotheism. This they did by incorporating him into a new figure they called Moses, who had never known the first Moses. This restoration, however, came at a cost to the truth, which had become "historical" rather than "material" truth (Freud, 1939). Another explanation for the repetition compulsion was put forward by Freud through his elaboration on theory of drives, and the introduction of the death drive.

The concept of the uncontrollable need to revisit painful events, has wide implications for the function of memory in the consulting room and the place of historical construction of truth in current psychoanalytic practice.

Bohleber (2007) argues that in some clinical situations, in PTSD for example, we find that memory no longer functions as helping toward integration and recovery. Rather, these patients live in a perpetual state of the past being relived in the present as if time had been frozen, and as if they never moved from the instance when the trauma occurred. The remembering, puts the patient in a state of re-traumatization.

In these clinical situations, Bohleber maintains, memories cannot be transformed merely by being retrieved and re-lived by the patient. They become like a foreign element in the psyche, where reality and phantasy are interwoven. What is required, is a reconstruction alongside recollection within a psychoanalytic relationship. In a therapeutic context, piecemeal historization can take place in which, crucially, traumatic facts need to be disentangled from unconscious phantasy.

There is, then, according to Bohleber, a place for reconstruction as an essential element of transformation in clinical practice. This, in cases of traumatization where the therapeutic task consists of helping to establish historical facts which are distinct from and free of the confusion between reality and unconscious feelings such as shame and guilt, that exacerbate the patients' suffering.

> Discovering the reality of the trauma and its associated affects – namely, its historicization, however fragmentary or approximate… Fantasy and traumatic reality are thereby disentangled and the ego acquires an alleviating context of understanding… . When such a reconstructive interpretation succeeds, patients often speak of astonishing improvements in their condition.
>
> Leuzinger-Bohleber & Bohleber, 2016, p. 65

This discussion highlights that historicization of trauma, unless sensitively done, can be a knife edge. It can give patients a sense of knowledge about themselves that can lead to integration and security. On the other hand, it can be another occasion of the compulsion to repeat, if remembering in and of itself is the objective. The difference in the phenomenology of traumatic distress remembered as either damaging or recuperative, I think, lies in the context in which the memory surfaces and, especially, how it is responded to. That is, whether recollection leaves the patient with an experience of being alone, in the same place as before, or whether historization is done within a containing analytic relationship, and in the context of an appropriate interpretive response (Bohleber, 2007).

The Restorative Effects of Memory in Literature and in *Moses and Monotheism*

In *Moses and Monotheism* Freud reflects on the process of recollection as a product of the undoing of repression. Earlier, in 1915 he wrote:

> there is no lifting of the repression until the conscious idea, after the resistances have been overcome, had entered into connection with the unconscious memory-trace.
>
> (pp. 175–176)

And, he believed, that for remembering to be effective in the process of psychic change, it needs to be felt and experienced, rather than just known or verbalized:

> To have heard something and to have experienced something are in their psychological nature two quite different things, even though the content of both is the same.
>
> (Ibid., p. 176)

This need for re-living a memory, for it to have a proper restorative effect, has also been demonstrated in literature.

In Chekhov's "In the cart" Marya is on a journey. She travels back to the little town where she lives and works, a nondescript outpost in the Russian countryside, having visited another small town where she bought some provisions. The journey has a symbolic meaning. It is a metaphor for a complex emotional process Marya is internally engaged with. It has been 13 years since she left Moscow, following the traumatic loss of her parents and her home. During the 13 year period she has lived in a psychological limbo, having erased Moscow and her past life from her memory; not allowing herself any remembrances that would cause her to re-experience the pain and conflicts surrounding the traumatic departure to the place where she was now living.

Marya's 13 years in the wilderness of a Russian outpost, and in her own inner life, can be described as her "latency" period that followed the repression of her trauma. It is similar to the story of the Jewish migration in the deserts of Egypt for a very long time, having forgotten the killing of their first leader Moses. On the long "latency" route, the Jews have also experienced various trials, until the memory of Moses has re-emerged.

On her way back to the town where she works and lives, Marya has a number of encounters which give her opportunities to recollect her past. These are initially rejected, until gradually she is ready for the memory of the past life to surface.

Then, as Chekhov's story progresses along an acutely observed psychological narrative, in a way similar to Freud's narrative in *Moses and Monotheism*, the time has come for Marya to reconnect. The barrier to her forgotten past is removed, just as she stands in front of train tracks fence by the station, and the barrier is being lifted. She has an extraordinary experience of seeing her (dead) mother waiting on the train station platform:

> Her mother! What a resemblance! Her mother had just such luxuriant hair… And with amazing distinctness, for the first time in those thirteen years, there rose before her mind a vivid picture of her mother, her father, her brother, their flat in Moscow… she felt as she had been then, young, good-looking, well-dressed, in a bright warm room among her own people. A feeling of joy and happiness suddenly came over her… she pressed her hands to her temples in an ecstasy, and called softly, beseechingly: "Mother!"

In her mind's eye Marya has seen her mother brought back to life, after a long time of being forgotten (Freud's "yawning gap" in *Moses and Monotheism*). Her now idealized childhood, before the trauma, has reworked itself into her consciousness. This experience, as the continuing story will show, will have a significant restorative effect on the way Marya will relate to others, with hopeful implications for her future.

Literary fiction, which brings to light essential aspects of the human condition, is not unlike the imaginative construction highlighted in Freud's story of the Jews in *Moses and Monotheism*, which also benefits from the freedom of subjectivity, and creativity. However, the difference between this and current psychoanalytic practice lies in the fact of it being seen as a two person's creation, in which both parties of the dyad affect each other, and to which story they contribute from their mutual subjectivities.

Historical Truth in the Intersubjective Field

In applying aspects of the archaeological construction model to *Moses and Monotheism*, Freud assumed a neutral relationship between the archaeologist and his find. Contemporary psychoanalysis, however, has put the analogy of impartiality into question. Objectivity in the relationship between the finder and the find, as in the archaeological model, had been contested.

Discoveries in other fields of knowledge, for example quantum physics, have thrown new light on the interdependence between the observer and the observed. Namely, what is being studied does not stay static during the investigation; it is transformed by being explored. There is no such thing as discovering a virgin island. The minute people set foot on the island to explore it, it is no longer "virgin." In other words, the very act of being present, witnessing, and noting impacts on what is being investigated.

This raises a question on the uncovering of historical truth in the intersubjective field, to which both parties of the analytic dyad contribute. In the clinical example quoted above the patient's historical recollection of the very significant onset for him changed over time, in line with the evolving transference relationship with his analyst. It was as though the patient's history was written and re-written, to accommodate his particular state of object relatedness at each instant of the telling.

This example accords with Freud's (1939) own view, put forward in *Moses and Monotheism*, on elements of subjectivity in the narration of historical truth:

> To begin with it had no scruples about shaping its narratives according to the needs and purposes of the moment… .
>
> (p. 68)

Freud provided ample evidence for the re-modeling of the story of Moses so as to rationalize an emerging need at a contemporary stage, following a long gap, that nevertheless required a reckoning with the past.

Bion (1970) elaborated on "the needs and purposes of the moment," by explicating on the concept of reasoning in general, which he saw as being secondary to affect. He thought that what seemed like a reasoned accounting of history was actually done in the service of emotions, and so as to explain experience.

"Reason is emotion's slave and exists to rationalize emotional experience. Sometimes the function of speech is to communicate experience to another; sometimes it is to miscommunicate experience to another" (p.1).

Following the Bionian insight into the function of language, there are observations of clinical situations where experience itself has been obliterated and is unavailable for representation, nor speech. To account for that, Bion (1992) introduced his radical idea that the primary analytic task can be converse to that of "making the unconscious conscious." Rather, patients in primitive psychotic states, need to be helped to establish unconscious functions in the first place, functions which neurotic patients can attain by the use of repression for example. In other words, they need assistance in developing the capacity to dream. The clinical use of the intersubjective field is of particular value in promoting this kind of transformation during the treatment of primitive states. The analyst can dream the patient, and, I would argue, ***for*** the patient for a while, lending his/her own psychic capacity for the patient to utilize. Narration of the patient's history would therefore be subjectively influenced by the presence of the analyst, and contributed to by the analyst's own unconscious historical truth (Collins, 2021).

Consequently, the dynamics and function of memory and historical construction in the intersubjective field, has evolved. From that of Freud, who would talk to patients *about* their early memories and present them with a *probable* construction of their past, to contemporary theory of practice, in which construction is viewed as being *subjectively co-created through the analyst's reverie*:

> I view reverie as an unconscious *construction* of patient and analyst who together create an unconscious third subject (the *analytic third*) who is the dreamer of reveries, which are experienced by patient and analyst through the lens of their own separate (conscious and unconscious) subjectivities... .
>
> (Ogden, 2017, p. 6)

With an increased use of analysts' observation of their own countertransference, emphasis in contemporary psychoanalysis has largely shifted to understanding the patient's unconscious communication via the analyst's unconscious. Therefore, the deployment of moments of "now" alive with affect, has been developed as the staging platform for understanding the past. Brown (2019) and Birksted-Breen (2019) have explored pathways to the analyst's unconscious through countertransference dreams, jokes, and through the analyst's soma. Collins (2020) also views other clinical phenomena such as enactments, the so-called "mistakes" by analysts, as additional pathways from the patient to the analyst's unconscious. These channels to the analyst's unconscious are ways of communicating, in the intersubjective field, early unrepresented and often un-experienced material.

Conclusion

Memory has been a corner stone of psychoanalytic investigation since Freud discovered it as the vehicle for recovery. While the phenomenology of historical recollection has subsequently been explored for its mutability and subjective vagaries, with some contemporary modifications of technique, it has retained its value as a pivotal restorative asset for patients.

In *Moses and Monotheism* Freud has re-established the psychological intensity and depth of memory, and showed the applicability of this psychoanalytic principle to group psychology, religion and other cultural field. He also explored the malleability of the notions of memory and historical construction, to the extent of asserting that psychotic beliefs too contain grains of historical truth. He demonstrated how assertions on truth about the past are contingent on the needs of a contemporary time. The present being a moment of "now," is suffused with unconscious affective needs, from which viewpoint patients remember and recount the past. Truth has many qualifications; it can be materially objective, but it can be subjective, and historically constructed to avoid uncomfortable conflict, the killing of the father figure in *Moses and Monotheism* being a prime example. Psychoanalysts have coined the term of "psychic truth." This is a truth of a particular quality, which reflects the temporality as well as the subjectivity of truth in historical memory. It is a truth of a unique kind, discovered only through the psychoanalytic process; the exploratory journey of an analytic dyad whose unconscious minds and inner lives jointly remember and create their own historical truth in an analytic field, so that psychic pain can be put in context, understood, and integrated. Memory of early life and its narration therefore remain seminal to clinical practice.

There are special implications for analytic practice regarding memory, in cases of trauma and primitive mental states, with their attendant aspects of non-representation and a severely impoverished unconscious. In these situations, the role of the analyst's unconscious countertransference is distinctive, in receiving communications from the patient and in offering recuperative understanding.

References

Bion, W. R. (1956). Development of schizophrenic thought, *International Journal of Psychoanalysis*, 37: 344–346.

Bion, W. R. (1959). Attacks on linking, *Int. J. Psychoanal.*, 40: 308–315.

Bion, W. R. (1962). The psycho-analytic study of thinking, *International Journal of Psychoanalysis*, 43: 306–310.

Bion, W.R. (1970). *Attention and Interpretation: A Scientific Approach to Insight in Psycho-analysis and Groups, The Complete Works of W. R. Bion*, Vol VI, pp. 221–330. London: Karnac Books, 2014.

Bion, W. R. & Green, A. (2005). Cogitations, *L'anneé Psychanalytique Internationale 2005*:233–241.

Birksted-Breen, D. (2019). Pathways of the unconscious: When the body is the receiver/instrument, *International Journal of Psychoanalysis*, 100: 1117–1133.

Bohleber, W. (2007). Remembrance, trauma and collective memory: The battle for memory in psychoanalysis, *Int. J. Psycho-Anal.*, 88(2): 329–352.

Bohleber, W. & Leuzinger-Bohleber, M. (2016). The special problem of interpretation in the treatment of traumatized patients, *Psychoanal. Inq.*, 36(1): 60–76.

Brown, L. J. (2007). On dreaming one's patient: Reflections on an aspect of countertransference dreams. *Psa Q*, 76: 835–861.

Brown, L. J. (1985). On concreteness, *Psychoanal. Rev.*, 72(3): 379–402.

Brown, L. J. (2019). *Transformational Processes in Clinical Psychoanalysis: Dreaming, Emotions and the Present Moment*, International Psychoanalytical Association. Psychoanalytic Ideas and Applications Series, Edited by G.Legorreta. London: Routledge.

Chekhov, A. (1919). In the cart. Translation: The Executors of the Estate of Constance Garnett. Granta Publications, London.

Collins, S. (2015). The voice behind the couch: whatever happened to the blank screen? in Bandler-Bellman, D, and Arundale, J. (Eds), *Interpretive Voice: Responding to Patients*. Karnac, London.

Collins, S. (2020). Psychic time as occasion for enactment, *The International Journal of Psychoanalysis*, 101.3: 436–455.

Collins, S (2021). Infantile aspects in analysts' enactments and changes in the setting. Paper given at the 52nd International Psychoanalytic Association Congress (online).

Eliot, T. S. (1935). Burnt Norton, The Four Quartets. In: *T.S. Eliot Collected Poems 1909–1962*, p. 177. London: Faber and Faber.

Freud, S. (1901b). *Psychopathology of Everyday Life*. London, 1950; New York, 1952; Standard Ed.

Freud, S. (1910a). *Five Lectures on Psychoanalysis*. London, 1950; New York, 1952; Standard Ed.

Freud, S. (1912–1913). *Totem and Taboo*. London, 1950; New York, 1952; Standard Ed.

Freud, S. (1915). *The Unconscious*. London, 1950; New York, 1952; Standard Ed.

Freud, S. (1920). *Beyond the Pleasure Principle*. London, 1950; New York, 1952; Standard Ed.

Freud, S. (1938). Constructions in analysis. *Int. J. Psycho-Anal.*, 19: 377–387.

Freud, S. (1939). *Moses and Monotheism: Three Essays*. London, 1950; New York, 1952; Standard Ed.

Levine, H. (2021). On the necessity of failure, Inaugural lecture, The Debbie Bellman Memorial Lecture, British Psychoanalytic Association, London (online).

Ogden, T. H. (1994). The analytic third: Working with intersubjective clinical facts, *Int. J. Psycho-Anal.*, 75:3–19.

Ogden, T. (2017). Dreaming the analytic session: A clinical essay, Psa. Q. 86:

Spence, D. (1982). On some clinical implications of action language. *Journal of the American Psychoanalytic Association*. 30:169–184.

Winnicott, D. W. (1945). Primitive emotional development, *Int. J. Psycho-Anal.*, 26: 137–143.

Winnicott, D. W. (1969). The use of an object, *Int. J. Psycho-Anal.*, 50: 711–716.

Winnicott, D. W. (1974). Fear of breakdown, *Int. R. Psycho-Anal.*, 1: 103–107.

Editor's Introduction to Chapter 6

Lawrence J. Brown

In this chapter, Sara Boffito explores Freud's hesitations in publishing *Moses and Monotheism*. The subtitle of this book, *Three Essays*, focuses on the three components that comprise this last book by Freud: two essays that were first published in *Imago* (1937) when he was still living in Vienna and a third that was published in 1939 after he had emigrated to London. It was this third portion of *Moses and Monotheism*, conceived when he was still in Austria, that Freud was most hesitant to publish because it would have been deemed heretical by the Catholic Church which provided an umbrella of relative safety from the Nazis. After months of anguish awaiting permission to relocate to the United Kingdom, Freud was finally in an environment sufficiently safe for completing the publication of all three chapters under the title of *The Man Moses: An Historical Novel*.

Boffito's research into the origins of *Moses and Monotheism* is impeccable as evidenced in her use of Freud's metaphor to describe his uncertainty of the book's future which "appears like a dancer balancing on the tip of one toe" (Freud, 1939, p. 58). This chapter is further enriched by her inclusion of Yerushalmi's (1989) translation of the unpublished preface to an earlier (1934) version of *Moses and Monotheism*. Yerushalmi's discussion introduces the notions of *historical truth* which aims at conveying an accurate depiction of a period in history that differs from a biographical study of an individual, such as Moses, and that

> nothing available concerning Moses can be called trustworthy. It is a tradition… revised several times and… closely interwoven with the religious and national myths of the people.
>
> (Ibid., p. 279)

Ultimately, Boffito describes how the final title of the book about Moses came to him: *The Man Moses, a Historical Novel* which brought together some contradictory ideas that he had been previously challenged to integrate.

DOI: 10.4324/9781003272045-12

Boffito introduces Freud's distinction between poetic license and historical truth which is linked with a hybrid view of Freud as an author: there is the Dr. Freud, the scientist who has written carefully thought-out treatises on psychoanalysis and related topics and Freud the author of imaginative works such as *Moses and Monotheism*. In this regard, she quotes Freud's letter (May 12, 1934, p. 77) to Arnold Zweig:

> we touch here on the problem of poetic license versus historical truth.... Where there is an unbridgeable gap in history and biography the writer can step in and try to guess how it all happened.

6 The Mule and the Dancer

Freud, Moses, and the Dilemma of the Hybrid

Sara Boffito

The edition we know of *Moses and Monotheism* has a subtitle, indeed a definition: *Three Essays*. Freud is referring to the fact that the book, which was released in 1938, is composed of two essays that appeared on "Imago" in 1937 and a third essay preceded by two Prefatory notes, both dated 1938. In them, Freud explains the reasons that had kept him from publishing the volume until then. The first of the two warnings is prior to March 1938, when Freud was still in Vienna. He wrote it "with the audacity of one who has little or nothing to lose" (Freud, 1939, p. 54). The tone is both heroic and resigned, with a hint of grandiosity. Freud, as we shall see, cannot refrain from writing about Moses but, living in a Catholic country where the Church is somehow protecting the Jews, he feels it necessary that a work which "leads us to a conclusion which reduces religion to a neurosis of humanity" (Freud, 1939, p. 55) must

> be preserved in concealment till some day the time arrives when it may venture without danger into the light, or till someone who has reached the same conclusions and opinions can be told: "there was someone in darker times who thought the same as you!"
>
> (Freud, 1939, p. 56)

A few months later, by now in London, where, after the invasion of Austria by the Nazis, he has found "freedom and safety," Freud ventures to bring the last portion of his work "before the public" (ibid.). Here he shares with readers the "*internal* difficulties" (Freud, 1939, p. 58) and obstacles to the publication of *Moses and Monotheism*. "I feel uncertain in the face of my own work; I lack the consciousness of unity and of belonging together which should exist between an author and his work" (Freud, 1939, p. 58). He confesses and describes his own uncertainty in these words: "This book, which takes its start from the man Moses, appears like a dancer balancing on the tip of one toe" (ibid.).

In the following pages I will try to follow the hesitations and also the virtuosities of this balancing dancer, without entering deeply into the dense and complex content of the Freudian text and of the mosaic

DOI: 10.4324/9781003272045-13

controversy. Instead, I follow the book's destiny and the ambivalence that Freud, old and troubled by the events of history, confesses so clearly as a lack of consciousness of unity between author and work. My hypothesis is that it is precisely in the folds of this incomplete adherence that one of the most valuable and unexpectedly contemporary fruitful aspects of this volume nests.

Out of the Half-Gloom of the Interior

We know that Freud's early interest in the figure of Moses resulted in obsession. He recognizes Moses as the "unlaid ghost" (Freud, 1939, p. 103) who, as he confesses to Lou Salome, "has pursued me throughout the whole of my life" (letter of January 6, 1935, p. 205). Following Freud's editorial relationship with Moses as a character, we already find evidence of this in the magnificent, small book, *The Moses of Michelangelo* (1914), in a "nonanalytical child" with whom Freud's relationship was "something like that to a love child" (as he writes to Edoardo Weiss in 1933, on the occasion of the Italian translation of the text, [p. 416]). The "nonanalytical child" is born during a journey to Rome in the company of Ferenczi in 1912, from days spent hypnotized by the statue of San Pietro in Vincoli, trying to solve the enigma enclosed in those shapes and expressions. It is equally true that such obsession – and identification – has always been accompanied by a combination of awe and sense of modesty. In the preface to *The Moses of Michelangelo*, Freud writes: "[I] have essayed to support the angry scorn of the hero's glance! Sometimes I have crept cautiously out of the half-gloom of the interior as though I myself belonged to the mob upon whom his eye is turned" (Freud, 1914a, p. 213).

On one hand, Freud is identified with the stern hero who leads a people to the conquest of new territories, as shown by the letter to Jung of January 17, 1909 in which he writes "if I am Moses, then you are Joshua" (Freud, 1909a, p. 196) and in another letter to Ferenczi of October 17, 1912. In that letter, he describes his dark mood, "According to my mood, I would sooner compare myself with the historical Moses than with the one by Michelangelo, which I interpreted" (Freud, 1912, p. 213). He refers to the character of a man that "had a hasty temper and was subject to fits of passion" (ibid., p. 233).

On the other hand, the editorial destiny of that first nonanalytical child is also marked by a lack of belonging between author and work: *The Moses of Michelangelo* appears on "Imago" in 1914 in anonymous form; Freud answers to Abraham, who insists that he assume the authorship, that the choice of anonymity is due to a mixture of "pleasantry" and "shame" (1914b, p. 228) – shame that he would feel also about himself from the merciless comparison with the austere and unreachable father Moses. The essay is accompanied by a note in which the editors explain that the article was accepted on an exceptional basis: "Although this paper does not, strictly speaking, conform to the conditions under which contributions are accepted for publication in this Journal, the editors have decided to print it, since *the author*, who is personally known to them, moves in psycho-analytic circles, and since his mode of thought has in point of fact a certain resemblance to the methodology of psycho-analysis" (p. 211, footnote 1, my italics).

This nonanalytical child was later acknowledged by Freud in 1924, when it seems that Freud's love for this text was so special precisely because it was colored by ambivalence, so much so that he invented, in the note just quoted, another author, known in the psychoanalytic circle, who would claim authorship.

The Blemish of Error

More than 20 years after his journey to Rome, Freud returned to reflect on Moses, and again, with much ambivalence, he would bring to light a nonanalytical child – a hybrid literary genre.

I am referring to an early version of *Moses and Monotheism*, which Freud completed in 1934 and never meant to publish. Probably it would not have been such a different book from the one that would come out in 1938. Freud had conceived of three chapters that would follow the argument that Moses, an Egyptian prince, had invented the Jew. The fundamental difference is in the title: "The Man Moses. A Historical Novel."

I am including here the entire unpublished preface to this first version, dated August 9, 1934, in the English translation reported in 1989 in the *International Journal of Psychoanalysis* by J. H. Yerushalmi:

> As the sexual union of horse and donkey produces two different hybrids, the mule and the hinny, so the mixture of historical writing and free invention give rise to different products which, under the common designation of historical novel, sometimes want to be appreciated as history, sometimes as novel. For some of them deal with people and events that are historically familiar, but they do not aim at reproducing them faithfully. They derive their interest, in fact, from history, but their intent is that of the novel; they want to sketch moving portrayals and to affect the emotions. Others among these literary creations function in quite the opposite way. They do not hesitate to invent persons and events in the hope of achieving an especially adequate description of the particular character of a historical period through such means, but first and foremost they aspire to historical truth despite the admitted fiction. Still others manage to a large extent in reconciling the demands of artistic creation with those of historical fidelity. How much fiction, contrary to the intentions of the historian still creeps into his presentation, requires little further comment!

> When I, however, who am neither a historian nor an artist, introduce one of my works as a historical novel, this term must allow for yet another definition. I have been trained to the careful scrutiny of a certain domain of phenomena. To me fiction and invention are easily associated with the blemish of error.
>
> My immediate purpose was to gain knowledge of the person of Moses, my more distant goal to contribute thereby to the solution of a problem, still current today, which can only be specified later on.
>
> A character study requires reliable material as its basis, but nothing available concerning Moses can be called trustworthy. It is a tradition coming from one source, not confirmed by any other, fixed in writing only in a later period, in itself contradictory, certainly revised several times and distorted under the influence of new tendencies, while closely interwoven with the religious and national myths of a people.
>
> One would be entitled to curtail the attempt as hopeless, were it not that the grandeur of the figure outweighs its elusiveness and challenges us to renewed effort. Thus one undertakes to treat each possibility in the text as a clue and to fill the gap between one fragment and another according to the law, so to speak, of least resistance, that is-to give preference to the assumption that can claim the greatest probability. That which one can obtain by means of this technique can also be taken as a kind of historical novel, since it has no proven reality, or only an unconfirmable one, for even the greatest probability does not coincide with the truth. Truth is often very improbable, and factual evidence can only in small measure be replaced by deductions and speculations.
>
> (Yerushalmi, 1989, p. 379)

In this unpublished preface, Freud proposes a twofold definition of the literary genre that this story, which had the urgency to be told. Yet, Freud cannot even manage to choose between the two hybrids – the mule and the hinny – placing himself in a third position, a somewhat clumsy and not entirely clear one, frightened by the shadow of the "blemish of error." He concludes with words of incredible modernity that seem almost contradicting the theoretical arguments about the value of historical truth that punctuate the book. In fact, he speaks of an "unconfirmable" reality that can at best approximate probability, or verisimilitude, not truth. It is a dilemma that runs through the entire book: The one concerning the possibility of authorizing oneself as a 'writer of verisimilitude' or as a novelist, which is particularly surprising since, throughout the text, we find it alternating with "a presentation of the theory of the traumatic origin of the neuroses so directly linked to the historical reality of the trauma as to recall, in some senses, the pre-psychoanalytic theories of *Studies on Hysteria*." (Barale, 1990, p. 897) – as Francesco Barale observes in a paper dedicated to the concept of trauma and historical truth in *Moses and Monotheism*.

We find in this indefinability of the genre – and especially in the choice not to publish, "The Man Moses" as a 'Historical Novel' – the same reluctance that, on the occasion of the publication of *The Moses of Michelangelo*, had driven Freud to resort to that *other author*, a non-analytical one, to whom he had attributed the authorship of the text.

Is this *other author* perhaps Freud the novelist? Who else would have found in Moses an object of research and obsession, but also of creativity and freedom?

A Complicated Fellow

Freud, orphan of Fliess, this time elects Arnold Zweig[1] as the privileged interlocutor of his dilemmas as a writer. In a letter addressed to him on May 8, 1932 – the answer to a sort of love declaration by his writer friend who, from Palestine, contemplated the Master's photo laid on his desk and imagined Freud in his Vienna home, admiring his resistance as a Jew who "has not run away" and told him about his writing projects around the Jewish theme (letter of May 1, 1932, p. 37). There, we find Freud for the first time struggling with ambivalence about the controversy concerning the origins of the Jew – a snapshot of that historical tragic moment, divided between persecution and the Zionist dream, but at the same time an example of how humanity universally needs to build and cultivate a myth of the origins. He writes:

> Palestine has produced nothing but religions, sacred frenzies, presumptuous attempts to conquer the outer world of appearances by the inner world of wishful thinking. And we hail from there (although one of us considers himself a German also, the other doesn't), our ancestors lived there perhaps for half, perhaps a whole, millennium (but this also only perhaps), and it is impossible to say how much of the life in that country we carry as heritage in our blood and nerves (as is mistakenly said). Oh, life could be very interesting if only one knew and understood more about such things! But the only things we can be sure of are our feelings of the moment!
>
> (Freud, 1932, pp. 411–412)

Already in these associations to his friend's journey we can detect in Freud the temptation to follow his own speculative imagination. He is hindered by the awareness – recalled in the preface to the Historical Novel – that one can be sure of almost nothing. It is as if he is afraid to overstep the mark, to reveal himself too much as a writer.

Interestingly, as early as 1930, the Italian writer and provocative futurist and visionary, Giovanni Papini perceived these characteristics in Freud when he narrated an imaginary meeting of the Master with "Gog" – an invented eccentric and bizarre character from an asylum. "Gog" wrote his memoirs from an asylum and delivered them to Papini himself. In this tale, Freud the character confesses to Gog: "Everyone believes that I care about the scientific character of my work and that my main goal is the cure of mental illness. This is an enormous misunderstanding that has lasted for too many years and that I have not been able to dispel. I am a scientist by necessity, not by vocation. My true nature is that of an artist. My secret hero has always been, since childhood, Goethe. I would have liked, then, to become a poet and all my life I have wanted to write novels" (Papini, 1930, p. 133). The conversation between the two characters ends with Freud's plea not to "spread his secret" (Papini, 1930, p. 135).

Papini's intuition appears even more bright if we remember that in 1930, the same year in which he imagines this irreverent conversation, Freud was awarded the Goethe Prize, on the basis that psychoanalysis has influenced the artists' conceptual world and somehow to compensate Freud, who had been "denied any official honorific recognition" as a scientist. In the speech (actually written by him but read by his daughter Anna because of his already precarious health) for this occasion that honors and surprises him, Freud approaches the theme of the "enigma of the wonderful gift that distinguishes the artist" contrasting it with the curiosity about his biography of those who worship him as if he were a hero: "a *powerful need* in us. We feel this very distinctly if the legacy of history unkindly refuses the satisfaction of this need" (Freud, 1930, p. 211, my italics).

It does seem that, in the last decade of his life, Freud was questioning the legitimacy of this powerful need to fantasize about both creativity of the artist and the origins of humankind, that he almost scoffs at having succumbed to a greedy curiosity about his idol Goethe. One almost smiles at this shyness in recognizing his own desire to be an artist, in the genius whose legacy is the revelation of the most unmentionable desires of humanity.

If we read the letters addressed to Arnold Zweig also as an internal dialogue, as always happens when we find an authentic interlocutor of our thought, we find there the confrontation of two contrasting and contradictory positions with which Freud himself was struggling. In 1934 – in a letter he summarizes his project as follows: "I soon found the formula: Moses created the Jew. And my essay received the title: *the Man Moses, a Historical Novel.*" Moreover, he confesses to his friend that he found himself writing *Moses the Egyptian* (what would become the first of the three essays that will make up the definitive edition of *Moses and Monotheism*) "in a time of relative freedom and at a loss to know what to do with my surplus leisure" contrary to what was his "original intention." The writing of that unusual text "has taken such a hold of me that everything else has been left undone" (letter of September 30, 1934b, p. 421).

And he would return to admit a few months later, "Moses won't let go of my imagination. I visualize myself reading it out to you when you come to Vienna, despite my defective speech." (Letter of May 2, 1935, p. 424.)

In the same epistolary exchange we find Freud expressing an extreme and uncompromising severity in front of one of his friend's projects, as if it were an indecency: Zweig consults him about the idea of writing "a novel about Nietzche's madness" (letter of April 28, 1934, p. 74) asking him also to request a contribution from Lou Salome.[2] Freud unreservedly declares his opposition to the project, stating that "we touch here on the problem of poetic license versus historical truth. I know my feelings on this point are thoroughly conservative. Where there is an unbridgeable gap in history and biography, the writer can step in and try to guess how it all happened. In an uninhabited country may be allowed to establish the creatures of his imagination." (Letter of May 12, 1934a, p. 77.)

On the one hand, Freud defines a boundary of legitimacy of the fantastic speculation, relegating it to very remote times and spaces, that authorizes himself to write *Moses and Monotheism*, that he compares to Thomas Mann's, *Joseph and His Brothers*, that he deeply loved. On the other hand, we cannot help but notice a certain stridor in Freud's moralistic severity if we compare it to the modernity of the considerations on verisimilitude, reality and truth with which he concludes his definition of the Historical Novel.

And it makes us smile even more, finding it even more jarring, if we compare these letters with those that Freud exchanged with the other Zweig writer, Stefan. Stefan Zweig not only had published a biography of Nietzsche in 1925 that would later be included in his trilogy dedicated to *The Struggle with the Demon*,[3] but also published a biography of Freud himself in 1931 In response to the publication, Freud does not hide a certain satisfaction, together with an almost too human narcissistic fragility, when we find him bothered by the biographer's insistence on his "*petit-bourgeois* correctness," because he states of himself: "The fellow is actually somewhat more complicated" (letter of February 7, 1931, p. 402).

The Other Author, the Novelist

A complex, complicated fellow. A character from whom, if only by scrolling through the letters around this subject, we see the emergence of a double – that *other author* who can shamelessly write and fantasize about the origins, inventing them, just as Moses invented the Jew.

Just in the pages of *Moses and Monotheism*, Freud wonders about men's imagination about distant eras of which we have only incomplete and blurred memories, observing that "this offers an artist a peculiar attraction, for in that case he is free to fill in the gaps in memory according to the desires of his imagination" (Freud, 1939, p. 71).

In 1909, in "Family Romances" – a short paper whose original title is *Der Familienroman Der Neurotiker*, where he uses the word *roman* (novel), the same as in *historischer Roman*, "Historical Novel" – Freud had traced in the neurotic "a quite peculiarly marked imaginative activity" that "starting roughly from the period before puberty, takes over the topic of family relations" (Freud, 1909b, p. 238). Thus, the child, "phantasy-builder" (Freud, 1909b, p. 239), tends to invent and narrate his own origin tale, driven by a thirst for knowledge and the impulse to achieve "the fulfillment of wishes" and "a correction of actual life" (Freud, 1909b, p. 238). Freud does the same, writing with the Moses, a sort of *Familienroman* of the Jews. Almost "contrary to his own intentions," Freud indulges the not merely infantile impulse of the "phantasy-builder" and makes of this book almost a hymn to creative imagination, inventing the story of a character who, in his narration, has even invented a whole people.

Following this thread, hidden in Freud's ambivalences, we can see the internal vicissitudes and obstacles to the publication of the "Historical Novel" as a sort of anticipation, a preconscious intuition by Freud, of one of the most fertile discourses of contemporary psychoanalysis. I am referring to the work of analysts who, after Bion, believe that waking dream thoughts and shared construction of stories, fantasies, and narratives are the royal road to analytic treatment.

The very act of dreaming, according to Grotstein, suggests that human beings must "be born with a propensity for story-telling, story-seeking, and story-responding, one that issues from the aesthetic vertex" (Grotstein, 2007, p. 275).

According to this approach, "the blemish of error," which Freud fears might dirty his scientific reasoning, becomes far less frightening, and indeed necessary. Such "narrative propensity," even a drive to narrate is necessary for the human being – defined as "story-teller" and "story requisitioner" – not to succumb to the anxiety caused by O, the thing itself. "The purpose of the story is to bind the anxiety created by O by transforming (transferring) it into a fictive but credible narrative structure that restores the subject's sense of cosmic causality and coherence" (Grotstein, 2007, p. 276).

This process, which Grotstein calls "narrativization" or "fictionalization," is certainly not indifferent to the search for truth; on the contrary, "the narrative function is able to preserve emotional truth [...], the raw data from O [...] become initially personified, as in children's cartoons, into personalized unconscious dreams and phantasies, which thereupon undergo a reconfiguration of story structure, a disarticulation of the object-linkages in the original cosmic event, and transvaluation of the emotional relationships to new unimportant entities for purposes of disguise" (Grotstein, 2007, p. 276).

If it is true, as Barale remarks, that in the pages of Moses, Freud seems to return to a theory of trauma linked to the historical reality that needs to be remembered, it is equally true that Freud's digressions around this book make us think of his urgency to write as an attempt to deal with the trauma that was going on at that time and that he, sharing with his friend Arnold Zweig the anguish for his own destiny and for that of all the Jews of Europe, suffered firsthand: the Holocaust. Here a later theory of trauma comes into play, the one of which Freud lays the foundations in *Inhibition, symptom and anxiety* (1926) and of which Baranger, Baranger, and Mom (1988) propose a further extension in the concept of "pure trauma." The authors first emphasize the need to move from the concept of trauma to that of "traumatic situation," which reactivates the primitive state of helplessness and presents itself as one of the vicissitudes of object relations. They also argue that "all forms of psychopathology as well as the 'normal' techniques of control are directed at avoiding the appearance of anxiety in this extreme form which is so primitive that we can only describe it in economic terms: rupture of the barrier, flooding by unmanageable quantities, complete helplessness" – "nameless dread" to use Bion's words (1962). It is an automatic anxiety that could be characterized as the initial trauma, "the pure trauma, meaningless, totally disruptive" (p.124). The tendency of human beings, in order to prevent as far as possible what might present itself as "pure trauma," is to give it a name:

> We demand that this trauma not be "pure" – purely economic – but instead a trauma that is inserted in a human history which, though it may be absurd, is at least a history. From this angle [...] the analytic process necessarily implies historicization. The brute event (accident, massacre, war, holocaust), in its effects on the individual who is our patient, cannot have meaning if it remains incidental and foreign. [...]
>
> *Psychoanalysis establishes itself against the pure trauma.* This does not mean that historization is an arbitrary process. As analysts, we cannot propose to anyone any history that is not his own. If at some point we try to substitute the "authentic" [...] for a piece of our own mind that is not adopted by the analysand with complete conviction, we are closing the process and inviting the subject to substitute a delusional conviction [...] with an insufficient history [...].
>
> We cannot function with the concept of a definitive history. We all know that analysands come with one history (sometimes remarkably poor) and "end" with a different, much richer history, with much subtler figures, moments of happiness and unhappiness, parents who are "good" and "bad" depending on moments and situations. The history we are left with can never be considered as an absolute term, as the "truth" substituted for the lie. This endlessness of the historicization process is what finally makes the analysis "interminable."
>
> (Baranger, Baranger, and Mom, 1988, pp. 124–125)

And, as Freud says in the aforementioned precious, unpublished preface to the "historical novel" of *Moses the Man*, it is what makes reality "unconfirmable." It seems to me that contemporary psychoanalysis can say out loud what Freud chose not to publish: it is what Nino Ferro masterfully summarizes every time he reminds us that the analyst's first task is a mourning of Reality (2021, 2017) and to foster in the patient an introjection of a narrative function, an inner "narrator," which allows, in the face of the most diverse emotional turbulence, to activate transformations toward thinkability (1999). We may then think of that *other author* as Freud's inner narrator, a personification of that necessary transformative function of reality. Looking at it from this implicit vertex, Freud's figure – even that of Freud as an analyst – becomes closer to the more contemporary figure of the wounded healer, of an analyst who faces the same mental operations and challenges that he helps the patient to recognize and overcome.

Similarly, the analyst who engages in analytic writing faces the same obstacles, the same demons that confront the writer. Thomas Ogden (2021) for this very reason compares the writing of any psychoanalytic essay to fiction writing, arguing that it is a form of autobiographical writing whereby the analyst puts his or her own private world on the page and that the act of writing engages the psychoanalytic writer in a process of being and becoming more fully himself or herself.

I would like to conclude by quoting some verses that Auden, in the same years in which Freud wrote *Moses and Monotheism*, dedicated to the "Novelist," whom the poet imagines as the holder of an almost boundless understanding of humanity, a figure at the same time sorrowful and discrete, that "must struggle out of his boyish gift and learn how to be plain and awkward," someone that "in his own weak person [...] Must suffer dully all the wrongs of Man." These are qualities that I feel are very close to those to which the contemporary psychoanalyst tries to achieve, and that I like to dedicate to that other author who – this is what I hope to have revealed – sometimes we can glimpse in Freud's text.

Notes

1 Arnold Zweig (1887–1968), German writer best known for his novel *Der Streit um den Sergeanten Grischa* (1927; *The Case of Sergeant Grischa*). In 1933 Zweig left Germany for Czechoslovakia. He later lived as an émigré in Palestine until 1948, when he moved to East Germany.

2 Freud will communicate the request to his beloved friend, telling her that he had already discouraged Zweig (letter of May 20, 1934) and she will answer with even more indignation: "It is absolutely out of the question that I should participate in this in any way. I cannot consider such a thing and the mere thought of it fills me with dismay. Please tell this to your correspondent in the strongest and

most final terms – moreover, how right you are to dissuade him altogether from his Nietzsche plan!" (letter of May 20, 1934, p. 203)

3 Zweig, S. (1939). *The Struggle with the Daemon: Hölderlin, Kleist, Nietzsche*. Pushkin Press, 2012.

References

Andreas-Salomé, L. (1934). Letter from Lou Andreas-Salomé to Freud, May 20, 1934. *Sigmund Freud and Lou Andreas-Salomé Letters* 89: 202–203.

Auden, W. H. (1940). *Another Time*. Faber & Faber, 2019.

Barale, F. (1990). Reflections on Freud's Moses (Trauma and History from the Last Freud to Us). *Rivista di Psychoanalisi* 36: 896–920.

Baranger, M., Baranger, W., & Mom, J. M. (1988). "The Infantile Psychic Trauma from Us to Freud: Pure Trauma, Retroactivity and Reconstruction." *International Journal of Psychoanalysis* 69: 113–128.

Ferro A (1999). *Psychoanalysis as Therapy and Storytelling*. Routledge, 2006.

Ferro, A. (2017). The Pleasure of the Analytic Hour. *The Italian Psychoanalytic Annual* 11:67–78.

Ferro, A. (2021). Like a Fish in Water. *Psychoanalytic Psychology* 38: 140–141.

Freud, S. (1909a). Letter from Sigmund Freud to C. G. Jung, January 17, 1909. *The Freud/Jung Letters: The Correspondence between Sigmund Freud and C. G. Jung* 41:195–197.

Freud, S. (1909b). *Family Romances*. The Standard Edition of the Complete Psychological Works of Sigmund Freud 9: 23–242.

Freud, S. (1912). Letter from Sigmund Freud to Sándor Ferenczi, October 17, 1912. *The Correspondence of Sigmund Freud and Sándor Ferenczi, Volume 1, 1908–1914* 25: 411–412.

Freud, S. (1914a). *The Moses of Michelangelo*. The Standard Edition of the Complete Psychological Works of Sigmund Freud 13: 209–238.

Freud, S. (1914b). Letter from Sigmund Freud to Karl Abraham, April 6, 1914. *The Complete Correspondence of Sigmund Freud and Karl Abraham 1907–1925* 52: 228–230.

Freud, S. (1926). *Inhibitions, Symptoms and Anxiety*. The Standard Edition of the Complete Psychological Works of Sigmund Freud 20: 75–176.

Freud, S. (1930). *The Goethe Prize*. The Standard Edition of the Complete Psychological Works of Sigmund Freud 21: 205–214.

Freud, S. (1931). Letter from Sigmund Freud to Stefan Zweig, February 7, 1931. *Letters of Sigmund Freud 1873–1939* 51: 402–403.

Freud, S. (1932). Letter from Sigmund Freud to Arnold Zweig, May 8, 1932. *Letters of Sigmund Freud 1873–1939* 51: 411–412.

Freud, S. (1933). Letter from Sigmund Freud to Edoardo Weiss, April 12, 1933. *Letters of Sigmund Freud 1873–1939* 51: 416.

Freud, S. (1934a). Letter from Sigmund Freud to Arnold Zweig, September 30, 1934. *Letters of Sigmund Freud 1873–1939* 51: 421–423.

Freud, S. (1934b). Letter from Sigmund Freud to Arnold Zweig, May 12, 1934. *Letters of Sigmund Freud and Arnold Zweig*. London: Tavistock, 1970.

Freud, S. (1934c). Letter from Freud to Lou Andreas-Salomé, May 16, 1934. *Sigmund Freud and Lou Andreas-Salomé Letters* 89: 202.

Freud, S. (1935). Letter from Freud to Lou Andreas-Salomé, January 6, 1935. *Sigmund Freud and Lou Andreas-Salomé Letters* 89: 204–205.
Freud, S. (1935). Letter from Sigmund Freud to Arnold Zweig, May 2, 1935. *Letters of Sigmund Freud 1873–1939* 51: 424–425.
Freud, S. (1939) *Moses and Monotheism: Three Essays*. The Standard Edition of the Complete Psychological Works of Sigmund Freud 23: 1–138.
Grotstein, J. (2007). *A Beam of Intense Darkness. Wilfred Bion's Legacy to Psychoanalysis*. London: Karnac.
Ogden, T. H. (2021). "Analytic Writing as a Form of Fiction." *Journal of the American Psychoanalytic Association* 69 (1): 221–223.
Papini, G. (1930). *Gog*. La scuola di Pitagora, 2017.
Yerushalmi, Y. H. (1989) Freud on the "Historical Novel": From the Manuscript Draft (1934) of Moses and Monotheism. *International Journal of Psychoanalysis* 70: 375–394.
Zweig, A. (1932) Letter from Arnold Zweig to Sigmund Freud, May 1, 1932. *The Letters of Sigmund Freud and Arnold Zweig* 84: 36–39.
Zweig, A. (1934). Letter from Arnold Zweig to Sigmund Freud, April 28, 1934. *The Letters of Sigmund Freud and Arnold Zweig* 84: 74–76.

Editor's Introduction to Chapter 7

Lawrence J. Brown

The analysis of a dream and its diverse associations leads the analyst in many directions: sometimes the tendrils of meaning seem to hang together and its "truth" is revealed to the analyst, corroborating his or her interpretations like the seamless fitting together of a jig-saw puzzle "from a confused heap of fragments" (Freud, 1923, p. 116). Earlier, in the *Interpretation of Dreams* (1900), he discussed the role of condensation in the dream's formation through a similar analogy:

> When the whole mass of these dream-thoughts [unconscious wishes] is brought under the pressure of dream-work, and its elements are turned about, broken into fragments and jammed together – almost like pack-ice...[1]
>
> (p. 312)

Rachel Blass argues that the agglomeration of a "confused heap of fragments" that are "jammed together – almost like pack-ice" and appear to confirm the veracity of the analyst's interpretation "does not mean that they are all true" (this volume). She connects this uncertainty to Freud's statement in *Moses* "that what is probable is not necessarily the truth and that the truth is not always probable" (Freud, 1939, p. 17.)

Blass observes that Freud's doubts about his assertions in *Moses* are unusually pronounced, even given that he typically questioned his own work, and he persevered in his belief that there was an historical truth behind his assertions in his book. She sheds light on Freud's own doubts about his convictions when he stated that

> No less than before, I feel uncertain in the face of my own work... But it is not as though there were an absence of conviction in the correctness of my conclusion.
>
> (1939, p. 58)

DOI: 10.4324/9781003272045-14

Blass takes the reader into Freud's thoughts about doubt and conviction, which he links with his earlier ideas about the return of the repressed (a subject discussed further in *Moses*), and from there to an illuminating account of his changing views on religion. The reader will no doubt find Blass' chapter thought provoking.

The author (LJB) thanks Dr. Rachel Blass for giving permission to reprint her 2003 paper, The Puzzle of Freud's Puzzle Analogy: Reviving a Struggle with Doubt and Conviction in Freud's *Moses and Monotheism*. *International Journal of Psychoanalysis*, 84: 669–682.

Note

1 "a large area of floating ice, usually occurring in polar seas, consisting of separate pieces that have become massed together," Collins English Dictionary.

7 The Puzzle of Freud's Puzzle Analogy

Reviving a Struggle with Doubt and Conviction in Freud's *Moses and Monotheism*

Rachel B. Blass

The Puzzle

Freud refers to an analogy of a jigsaw puzzle only three times throughout his published writings.[1] This puzzle analogy is best, and in fact almost exclusively, known from his use of it in his 1923 paper "Remarks on the theory and practice of dream-interpretation." There, Freud deals with the problem of corroborative dreams, that is, those dreams that confirm earlier analytic interpretations. Freud raises the question whether these dreams are not, in fact, the result of the analyst's suggestion. He explains that such doubt may arise not only in the patient, but in the analyst as well. It is here that Freud introduces a jigsaw puzzle. He writes:

> What makes him certain in the end is precisely the complication of the problem before him, which is like the solution of a jig-saw puzzle. A colored picture, pasted upon a thin sheet of wood and fitting exactly into a wooden frame, is cut into a large number of pieces of the most irregular and crooked shapes. If one succeeds in arranging the confused heap of fragments, each of which bears upon it an unintelligible piece of drawing, so that the picture acquires a meaning, so that there is no gap anywhere in the design and so that the whole fits into the frame – if all these conditions are fulfilled, then one knows that one has solved the puzzle and that there is no alternative solution
>
> (p. 116)

It would seem that Freud here maintains that when an interpretation allows for the meaningful coherence of the pieces of the dream into which it is fragmented in the course of the dream analysis, we have in our hands evidence of the truth of that interpretation. Or as Freud more assertively states, "there is no alternative solution."

DOI: 10.4324/9781003272045-15

A similar and rarely cited use of this analogy is found in Freud's 1896 paper "The aetiology of hysteria."[2]

This puzzle analogy is much cited within the literature. Relying primarily on the 1923 paper, numerous works have referred to the analogy and subjected it to careful study (e.g. Meissner, 1971; Rogers, 1981). As a rule, the analogy is considered to be a very important dimension of Freud's epistemological model, an informal reference to an underlying coherence theory of justification. While some have considered it an important stepping-stone to a kind of narrative approach to psychoanalysis (Steele, 1979), more common is a critical evaluation of the analogy as a problematic, limited form of justification (e.g. Spence, 1982; Blass, 2002, pp. 92–95). The main line of criticism is simply that interpretations may make sense of the fragments, but this does not mean that they are all true, that is, that they are indeed reflecting the unconscious wish or reality that the patient was expressing through his dream or through the other kind of material presented in analysis, as Freud indeed believed them to be.

This analogy, however, is not only potentially limited and faulty, it is also strikingly puzzling. Its puzzling nature emerges by taking note of the third and final instance in which Freud makes use of this analogy, albeit in a way very different from the only other two references to it. This is in the second part of his monograph on Moses, first published in 1937. In that part, entitled "If Moses was an Egyptian …," Freud writes about his hesitations regarding arguing publicly in favor of the implications arising from his hypothesis that Moses was an Egyptian. He maintained that these implications arose only from psychological probabilities and not from objective proof, and since they were of great importance, he felt that they (the implications) should not be presented without more secure foundations. The danger would be from the "critical assaults of the world around one" (1939, p. 17). It is here that he refers to his puzzle analogy once again. He writes:

> Not even the most tempting probability is a protection against error; even if all the parts of a problem seem to fit together like the pieces of a jig-saw puzzle, one must reflect that what is probable is not necessarily the truth and that the truth is not always probable
>
> (p. 17)

"What is probable is not necessarily the truth." Having just completed extensive work on the justification of Freud's dream theory I had occasion to read Freud's *Moses* and I was immediately struck by this statement. While numerous papers have taken Freud to task for relying on the notion that what coheres is true, here Freud himself states straight out that "what coheres may not be true, and coherence cannot be relied on as a form of justification." (This statement is neglected even by Strachey, who cross-references the puzzle analogy of 1896 and 1923, but leaves out the later reference to it (Freud, 1896, p. 205).

So here is the puzzle: how could Freud at one moment use the puzzle analogy to support the truth of his interpretations and at another, with the same sense of certainty and without any mention of a change of mind, point to the limitations of such an analogy as a source of support? It is in the attempt to answer this question that we gain both a better understanding of Freud's puzzle analogy but, more importantly a better understanding of the state of mind in which Freud was constructing his *Moses*, and, more specifically, with Freud's struggle with the feelings of doubt and conviction that arise as he searches for truth in that context. All these emerge from a closer look at some important dimensions of Freud's *Moses and Monotheism*, especially in the context of his broader theoretical framework. This closer look provides the missing pieces to the puzzle that we are now faced with. After laying out these missing pieces I will return to solve the puzzle. While each of these pieces deserves a much more extensive discussion, I will here present them in a rather concise form in order to reach some resolution of the puzzle within the context of this chapter.

The Centrality of Doubt and Conviction in *Moses*

One piece of the puzzle as to why Freud in *Moses* rejected the puzzle analogy has to do with the centrality of the issue of doubt and conviction throughout the book. In many of his writings Freud expresses doubt and uncertainty regarding his own work, and comments on the unfinished nature of his findings or their overly speculative basis (see Mahony, 1982, pp. 103–26). The nature of the doubt expressed in *Moses* is, however, outstanding. Not only does it consistently appear throughout the entire book, but it becomes a central issue. It is central as Freud reflects on the difficulties in the process of discovery, and it is central to what is being discovered. In *Moses*, Freud is doubtful as he makes new discoveries regarding the nature of doubt and its complement or opposite in this context, conviction. The doubts on the levels of personal reflection and subject of study seem to converge. Let me put forward just a few examples.

Freud ends his first essay on Moses with the following remark:

> We have seen that the first argument, based on his name, failed with many people to carry conviction. We must be prepared to find that this new argument, based on an analysis of the legend of exposure, may have no better success. It will no doubt be objected that the circumstances of the construction and transformation of legends are, after all, too obscure to justify a conclusion such as ours and that the

> traditions surrounding the heroic figure of Moses – with all their confusion and contradictions ... are bound to baffle every effort to bring to light the kernel of historical truth that lies behind them. I do not myself share this dissenting attitude but neither am I in a position to refute it.
>
> (1939, pp. 15–16)

The doubt and the conviction are there from the start. Freud puts forth an argument, notes that unfortunately it has failed to convince others – *others* will 'no doubt' object. But while attributing doubt to these others, Freud does not deny that there are good grounds for this doubt. And yet, despite the legitimate doubt and his inability to refute it, Freud expresses his conviction nevertheless. He *believes* that the truth behind the Moses story can be attained. He goes on to state that if "one allows oneself to be carried away by the ... arguments ... very interesting and far-reaching prospects are opened up" and here lies the value of his work. Is Freud here not suggesting that one should bracket doubt because of the value of the results? This would be a strange claim for Freud, who in the past rejected such lines of reasoning especially in the context of religion (1927), but more generally maintained that the value of one's assertions lies in the truths that they contain (Letter to Einstein, May 3, 1936, in E. Freud, 1960, p. 428).

He concludes the first essay with a decision to drop any further enquiry because, in the absence of more firm evidence, he will not be able to defend his findings from external critique (1939, p. 16).

As we know, Freud was soon to proceed with his second essay. In its course internal doubts do begin to come to the surface, and it is in this context that Freud mentions the puzzle analogy and how coherence of the pieces cannot protect from error.

Freud's solution to the mixture of doubt and conviction "which weigh as much with me today as they did before," is to go ahead with the conviction (p. 17). Without providing any new arguments for this move he indeed brackets the doubt (or, to use his own metaphor, puts the doubt outside the brackets of the present study) and decides to see where the questionable findings will lead. The title of the second essay clearly reflects this move: "If Moses was an Egyptian ..." (p. 17). The tentative phrasing continues throughout. But Freud is also careful to remind us of this, again pointing to his own awareness and perhaps growing uneasiness with the lack of adequate evidence. He writes (again with an initial concern with the external critic):

> I expect to be told that I have brought forward this structure of conjectures with too much positiveness, for which there is no basis in the material. This objection is, I think, unjustified. I have already laid stress on the factor of doubt in my introductory remarks: I have, as it

> were, placed that factor outside the brackets and I may be allowed to save myself the trouble of repeating it in connection with each item *inside* them.
>
> (p. 31)

After further exploring his hypothesis he repeats his concern with the certainty that he has expressed, now allowing the concern to shift from the doubts of others to his own doubts. Once again I am prepared to find myself blamed for having presented my reconstruction of the early history of the people of Israel with too great and unjustified certainty. I shall not feel very severely hit by this criticism, since it finds an echo in my own judgment (p. 41).

Aware of the weaknesses he decides to continue. As he asserts without explanation, "On the whole my predominant impression is that it is worth while to pursue the work in the direction it has taken" (p. 41). But the doubt now becomes more explicit. In the third essay he writes, for example, that "As regards *internal* difficulties [in contrast to the external ones] … No less than before, I feel uncertain in the face of my own work … [But it] is not as though there were an absence of conviction in the correctness of my conclusion" (p. 58).

As I have noted earlier, Freud's doubts and conviction seem to correspond to a major focus of the *subject* of Freud's study as well. A major concern is how we have conviction, "from what sources some ideas … derive their power to subject both men and peoples to their yoke" (p. 52, see also pp. 127–128). In a more specific sense, he wants to know how come the traditions that have shaped the Jewish people, and most notably their traditions regarding God and the relationship with him, have come to be accepted as true. But the broader question is how is it that beliefs that are not only unverified by reality but are also incompatible with it are not simply "listened to, judged, and perhaps dismissed, like any other piece of information from outside" (p. 101)? How come they arouse such compulsive conviction rather than a doubtful stance that would naturally arise from applying the constraints of logical thought?

As Freud loosens the constraints of his own logical thought and takes what he refers to as "a plunge" (p. 58) into the heart of his speculations regarding the history of the Jews, as he allows himself to "be carried away by the arguments," and at one point even suggests to the reader that we should "greatly tone down the strictness of the requirements in this study" (p. 105) because of its potential, one begins to wonder whether we are not witnessing in Freud himself, in the course of the writing of *Moses*, the very power of ideas which intrigued him in this study. Was he not being driven, to the neglect of material reality as he viewed it, by the force of an idea of which he was deeply, may we say, compulsively convinced? Was it not the knowledge that some truth is concealed within convictions of this kind that led him to continue to reinterpret the biblical text although he thought that "the distortion of a text resembles a murder' (strangely emphasizing in this analogy the ease of committing such an act and only the difficulty of concealing it)?

As Freud immediately shifts from doubt regarding the veridicality of his own reconstructions of the biblical story to the doubtful nature of the biblical story itself, as he shifts from his strong desire to follow through his questionable reconstruction to "the powerful tendentious purposes" that went into the writing of the Bible in the first place, resulting in the distortion of the truth, the convergence of the different levels of doubt and conviction is most striking (p. 41).

Freud's Theories of Doubt and Conviction

Having pointed out the central place of doubt and conviction in the writing and content of *Moses*, I turn now to describe Freud's theoretical formulations of the phenomena of doubt and conviction, formulations that are especially developed in the course of the *Moses* book. This is the second piece of the puzzle. The issue of Freud's theories of doubt and conviction has never been fully studied and deserves a more extensive review. However, here guided by my more limited aim of outlining the pieces necessary for resolving the puzzle that Freud presents us with, my presentation is brief and schematic.

It may be seen that Freud held two main kinds of theories related to doubt and conviction. These theories offer a psychoanalytic understanding of the dynamics that underlie these phenomena.

The first kind of theory is *drive-oriented*. One version of this kind of theory is of particular interest. It is described most clearly in Freud's explanation of his famous case of the Rat Man:

> The *doubt* corresponds to the patient's internal perception of his own indecision, which in consequence of the inhibition of his love by his hatred, takes possession of him in the face of every intended action. The doubt is in reality a doubt of his own love – which ought to be the most certain thing in his whole mind; ... A man who doubts his own love may, or rather *must*, doubt every lesser thing.
>
> (1909, p. 241)

When love is inhibited by hatred a person can no longer trust his own love and the consequence is indecision experienced as doubt. The other side of the coin is compulsion, which in the realm of ideas resembles conviction in terms of the experience. In this first theory compulsion is understood as "an attempt at a compensation for the doubt and at a correction of the intolerable conditions of inhibition to which the doubt bears witness" (p. 243).

To keep our puzzle in focus, it should be mentioned here that, in the context of the 1923 reference to the puzzle analogy, Freud is concerned with doubt in accordance with this theory. He mentions there that corroborative dreams are produced especially by doubters, implying that their indecision does not allow them to affirm the analyst's interpretation in a more direct way.

Freud's second kind of theory in the context of doubt and conviction is not concerned with the interplay of libidinal and aggressive drives, but rather with "the return of the repressed." Interestingly, its main exposition is to be found in *Moses and Monotheism*. Here the focus is on conviction. In a nutshell, conviction, according to this theory, is the experience that emerges when an idea that is presented for belief corresponds in some way to a deeply repressed memory or event. Powerful events leave permanent traces in the mind that are repressed and distorted. When at a later point one meets with (or creates) an idea that is a distorted reflection of these events, the idea will be accepted as true, in fact it must be, compulsively, believed. This is because of the resonance of the idea with the trace of the real event that is imprinted in the mind. Thus Freud explains that:

> When Moses brought the people the idea of a single god, it was not a novelty but signified the revival of an experience in the primaeval ages of the human family which had long vanished from men's conscious memory ... [but which] had left behind it in the human mind some permanent traces.
>
> (1939, p. 129)

Consequently, Moses's idea of a single God, although according to Freud, incompatible with reality, "*must* be believed" (p. 130). It corresponds with truth as permanently registered within the mind.

In this theory doubt is not the immediate complement of compulsive conviction. It would seem that one either is compelled to believe by the force of the memory traces of past events, or one has not been witness to past events that have left such forceful memory traces. But it may be suggested that Freud, both through his own affirmed atheism and through his theory of cure, maintained that it is possible to overcome compulsive conviction in this sense by turning more directly to material truth, to the actual reality that underlies the inner truths in their distorted form. Doubt here would then be a skeptical stance based on openness to, and concern for, material reality. In this formulation it is not so much a dynamically determined phenomenon as the overcoming of the dynamically determined phenomenon of conviction. So we have here two very different models of doubt and conviction, and I will suggest that these were playing into Freud's experience of doubt and conviction, which as we have seen were very central in the course of his writing.

Freud's New View of Religion

The third piece of the puzzle has to do with the new view of religion that Freud puts forth in *Moses and Monotheism*. My interest here is to emphasize only two points.

The first is that in *Moses and Monotheism* Freud shifts toward a much more positive view of religion than ever before. Indeed, religion continues to be referred to as a kind of neurosis, and as, in part, distortive and delusional. But now this is only a part. More than ever before Freud recognizes and stresses the positive developments made possible by religion. Through his focus specifically on the Jewish people (and perhaps also by distinguishing a religious elite within this people) he now speaks of religion in terms of advances in intellectuality, encouragement of sublimation, higher ethical aspirations. The higher psychical activities that emerge "help ... to check the brutality and the tendency to violence" (1939, p. 115). By introducing the spiritualized notion of God Moses, "set before men as their highest aim a life in truth and justice" (p. 50). The ideals that Freud here attributes to religion are the ideals that he himself held to be of the highest kind and the end of humanity – that is, if it is to succeed.

Freud himself was aware of this positive shift. In the postscript to *An Autobiographical Study* (written while he was preparing his *Moses and Monotheism*) he explains that, while in *The Future of an Illusion* (1927) he "expresses an essentially negative valuation of religion," later he "found a formula which did better justice to it ... granting that its power lies within the truth that it contains" (1935, p. 72). Lou Andreas-Salomé, with whom Freud corresponded regarding *Moses*, recognized this positive shift as well. In one response in January 1935, she writes to Freud that in contrast to his earlier use of the notion of the return of the repressed to denote neurotic processes, now "we are presented with examples of the survival of the most triumphant vital elements of the past as the truest possession in the present" (in Pfeiffer, 1966, p. 206).

Here we see that the positive developments that are now acknowledged, the power and vitality of religion, are intimately tied to the notion of its truth. This leads to the second point regarding Freud's new view of religion that I would like to stress – the close and complex relationship that Freud is now positing between religion and truth. Of course, Freud never completely dissociated the two. Ever since *Totem and Taboo* (1912–13), Freud openly claimed that at the basis of religious belief there lay a series of real historical events, and in *The Future of an Illusion* he argued that the believer, in his wishful fantasies of the existence of God, was re-experiencing a child–parent relationship that at one time did *in fact* exist. But in *Moses and Monotheism* there is a difference. Now Freud posits that at the heart of religion is not distortion, but truth. The truth is an early one, but not necessarily of an infantile kind that should be overcome by any mature adult. The powerful primaeval events that determine religious belief are now compared with other early impressions, not necessarily of a pathology-inducing kind, that later impact our character governing our actions, deciding our sympathies and antipathies, determining the choice of a love object "for which," Freud adds, "it is so frequently impossible to find a rational basis" (1939, p. 126). And just as one's loves need not be constantly reduced to their oedipal origins in order to live as a mature and rational being, so in this comparison it becomes unclear whether it is incumbent upon the believer to move beyond his belief in order to live maturely and rationally. With religious belief bringing in its course so many positive developments and at the heart expressing a truth, why not believe? While Freud does not himself ask this question as such, its presence is felt as he lists the virtues and truthful source of belief, and the question cannot be answered with the simple response that Freud offered on other occasions, that belief contradicts reality (1927, p. 32). It contradicts material reality as Freud knows it, but it may do so no more than does the lover's appreciation of his beloved (1915).

To take this point one step further, it may be suggested that Freud's reference at the very end of *Moses and Monotheism* to the evolution of Christianity is an expression of his doubt whether it is, in fact, possible to move closer to the material truth of the primal patricide than Judaism already allows for. The move toward this truth initiated by Paul, according to Freud, could not be borne and led to increased distortion and ultimately to culturally regressive steps from the perspective of Freud's monotheism (1939, p. 88).

In this more accepting view of the value, truth, and perhaps even necessity of religious belief, we see a dramatic shift away from Freud's more common position, which considers it primarily a reality-distorting teaching founded on an infantile wish for a protective father, which, in the service of truth, maturity, and cultural development, must be overcome (1927, p. 44). The value of this piece of the puzzle becomes apparent through its connection to the next one.

Freud's Struggle with a New Area of Reality

The fourth piece of the puzzle is Freud's struggle with a new area or kind of reality. Religion, as Freud was now understanding it, highlighted for him a dimension of reality that he was reluctant to fully recognize. Between the internal reality of fantasy and the actual material reality there lay religious belief, grounded in what he referred to as "historical truth," which did not correspond to material reality, but did not simply contradict it either. It was a truth impressed upon the mind, but beyond the mind's capacity to have ever comprehended it (1939, p. 126), and thus registered in the mind with distortions. Its source was a real external reality, but the impression was not equivalent to that reality either, reflecting in part the interaction with it, or the experience of it (p. 126).[3]

It is through this notion of truth that Freud describes a reality that stands beyond the objective factual claims of the propositions contained within beliefs and ideas, as well as beyond their inner wishful sources. Indeed, beliefs and ideas may be measured in terms of objective material reality and to the extent that they are shaped by the limitations of the mind or the power of wishes and desires they would, according to Freud, have to be regarded as delusional, as false (pp. 123, 129). But to the extent that they convey the great truths of "the earliest experiences of the whole of humanity" that return and find revived expression in our minds and in our lives, they also reflect a true reality, albeit not merely of an internal kind (p. 130). In other words, while the attempt to give conscious and ideational form to such powerful experiences of the past produces beliefs and ideas that as propositions regarding objective reality are false, they are nevertheless true to the past reality as it had originally been experienced and is now impressed upon the mind. In fact, they are, in a sense, *most* true to this reality; for when the expression of what was impressed upon the minds of men in primaeval times comes closest to the original experience and to the traces it left within, it stands at a distance from the material reality objectively perceived today. In this sense, such ideas, "distorted" in terms of material the objective factual claims of the propositions contained within beliefs and ideas, as reality, are "justified memor[ies]" in terms of this new kind of reality which Freud deals with here (p. 130).

To some degree, Freud was always aware of the existence of this third kind of reality (between internal and external), from his early seduction theories onward. Indeed, it may be argued that it was especially in these early seduction theories that Freud became aware of how the real external world impressed itself on the mind of the child in a way that could not be equated with the external stimulus, since the sexual nature of the stimulus was beyond what a child could possibly experience according to those early theories (Blass, 1992; Blass and Simon, 1994). But it is only here in *Moses and Monotheism* that there is an attempt to accept this reality as having a place of its own and not merely weigh and judge it in terms of inner wishes and external realities. It is not a drive or a simple memory or fact. Nor, as we have seen, is it necessary, or necessarily possible, to reduce it to either of these factors. For, as Andreas-Salomé explains, it is in the belief that the "most triumphant vital elements" have survived (in Pfeiffer, 1966, p. 206).

But Freud could not just give up reality in the common material sense of the term. In fact, he did not, and although, according to his theory, there is a compulsion for Jews to believe, he rejected the pious accounts of truth and history. Before the writing of *Moses and Monotheism* this rejection was very outright and straightforward. The choice was between reality and distortion, between what Freud referred to as his "God Logos," and infantile wishes (1927, p. 54). In *Moses*, however, where the advances in abstract thought, intellectuality, and truth became part and parcel of religious belief in its proper form, and belief essentially culture-enhancing, the battle between Logos and distortion could no longer be defined or played out as neatly as before.

In the place of this battle a struggle with this new kind of historical truth ensues. It finds expression in Freud's shifts between his persistent search for the material facts that lie at the source of religious belief and his repeated request that we, the readers, limit our constraints of reason, bracket our doubts, so that the findings, apparently valuable to Freud independently of their material truth (as historical truth itself is independently valuable), may be explored. This struggle also finds expression in his reference to the puzzle analogy to which I now return.

The Solution of the Puzzle

So now we have a small heap of fragments. In the following pages I will not try to make all the rough edges fit together, leaving no gaps or alternative solutions, but rather will merely outline one solution to the puzzle of the puzzle analogy which I have found to be convincing and valuable to the understanding of Freud and some of his major concerns.

To recall, the problem was that Freud in 1923 had applied the jigsaw puzzle analogy to argue that coherence is a source of certainty that one has arrived at the truth, a controversial position within the psychoanalytic literature. Then in *Moses* Freud uses the very same analogy to argue the opposite, namely, that coherence does not necessarily lead to truth.

When viewed in the light of Freud's ideas on certainty, doubt, truth, and reality, that he was both putting forth and directly and intensively experiencing especially in the context of *Moses*, as may be seen in the fragments that I have now set forth, this apparent contradiction becomes more coherent.

Freud's struggle with historical truth, as he understood it in *Moses and Monotheism*, on the one hand enhanced his doubt and on the other increased his conviction. On the one hand, he realized that the methods he applied in the past to gain certainty could not provide it here. Coherence may be indicating truth, but in this case it may be in the historical sense of the term, without ever revealing the material truth to which Freud was ambivalently aspiring. Material truth may, forever, lie beyond the reach of the historical truth that Freud may discover through the analysis of the lives of individuals and peoples. Freud at points feared this elusiveness of material truth, albeit through his fear of "critical assaults of the world around one" (1939, p. 17).

But, on the other hand, Freud now recognized a new source for his certainty, realizing both the strength of his conviction and, in a sense, and again in an ambivalent way, its legitimate grounds. That is, Freud now knew that the sense of conviction that he was experiencing (despite lack of sufficient evidence) may not be merely a pathological compensation for pathological doubt, but rather a reflection of a reality, albeit elusive and perhaps distorted. In this context it is important to see that the puzzle analogy, more than a strong epistemological statement may be a therapeutic one. It may be considered a statement on how to deal with the psychological phenomenon of doubt, rather than one on how to discover unquestionable truth. Thus in the 1923 reference Freud would be saying that the analyst's *experience* of doubt, his fear that he is forcing his interpretations upon the dreamer, determined, like the doubt of the dreamer himself, by a lack of trust in his own love, can be overcome by the *experience* of coherence.[4] The epistemological question of whether or not this coherence indicates that unquestionable truth has been attained would be another matter. But with the powerful sense of conviction and his new theory of conviction this therapeutic analogy has no place. In a sense Freud now became aware of the fact that he was being moved by a truth despite any doubt, and that he trusted the validity of this pressing truth, regardless of the fitting together of the pieces of a puzzle. Noting the lack of sufficient evidence for his conclusions, he confides to Andreas-Salomé that, "It suffices me that I myself can believe in the solution of the problem" (January 6, 1935, in Pfeiffer, 1966, p. 205). In sum, not only did the value of the puzzle analogy become more limited as Freud struggled with the new epistemological problems that arose from his growing concern with historical reality, but also, given the experience of conviction, which was now intermittently guiding Freud's work, the puzzle analogy became superfluous as a means for relieving feelings of doubt. Moreover, relief from doubt itself may have become an ambivalently desired aim, inasmuch as Freud himself was directly involved in the study of the meaning of doubt and its opposite, conviction.

It would seem that in *Moses* what was of greater value to Freud than fitting the pieces of the puzzle together was the attempt to do so (an attempt that I had the opportunity to share in while solving the puzzle that Freud's writing posed for me), for it is within the attempt, the struggle to fit the pieces together, that Freud encountered his conviction despite doubt in a truth that the puzzle could only point to.

Implications for Understanding the Nature of the Text of *Moses and Monotheism*

In the course of putting together the pieces of the puzzle new perspectives on some of Freud's ideas and concerns have been offered. Reference has been made to a therapeutic dimension of Freud's apparently epistemological statements, to a dramatic shift in Freud's attitude to religion, to connections between Freud's early fears of imposing his interpretations[5] and his later sense of doubt and certainty, etc. One other implication, which I will soon describe here, pertains to the issue of the basic nature of Freud's *Moses and Monotheism* (e.g. science, fiction, history, myth, etc.?). It is because of the close relationship between the process of solving the puzzle and my understanding of the nature of the book that I expand on this point in the present context.

The issue of the basic nature of the text of *Moses and Monotheism* has been subject to much debate. Grubrich-Simitis in her important in-depth study of the book suggests that its basic nature is, in fact, very multi-determined. She writes:

> It is many things all at once: psychology of religion; biblical criticism; fictional rewriting of a myth; a history of the formation of Freudian theory; a monograph on the genesis of individual and collective neurosis; a recapitulation of the theory of civilization; psychohistory; a political treatise; and a metaphorical autobiography.
>
> (1997, p. 60)

And indeed, many writers, Bible critics, historians, anthropologists, and psychoanalysts have at one time or another regarded the book in terms of these possibilities. Grubrich Simitis herself adds to this list her own central idea that the book may be regarded as a day-dream as well.

By working through the puzzle of Freud's puzzle analogy there evolves, alongside new understandings of the content of Freud's concerns in *Moses and Monotheism*, an alternate view of the book's very nature. This new view of the book takes into account the other kinds of understandings that have already been put forth, but also differs from them all in a fundamental way. To see how and why this is so, it is important first to recognize that all the existing theses regarding the nature of Freud's *Moses and Monotheism* may be divided along one important dimension: whether or not they view Freud as actually involved in a serious search for the truth regarding Moses as he apparently claims to be. As a rule, those who take his claim seriously (including those who do so temporarily for the sake of argument) regard the book as a terrible failure, producing an "arbitrary manipulation of dubious historical data," rather than scientific formulation (Yerushalmi, 1991, p. 2). Those who, on the other hand, reject Freud's claim, find value in the book by arguing that its blatant failure as science or history points to the presence of latent agendas of other kinds (Rice, 1990, p. 152; Yerushalmi, 1991, pp. 2, 35; Paul, 1994, p. 835, 1996, p. 223; Assman, 1997, p. 147; Bernstein, 1998, pp. 72, 87). They contend that Freud is not searching for truth in the sense of trying to discern and demonstrate statements about the history of ancient Egypt and Israel, or actual causes of human evolution, but rather through the framework of this historical endeavor is, in fact, giving expression to wishes, fantasies, dreams, speculations, myths and personal stances, beliefs, questions, and ideas on a range of issues and with a range of aims (personal, social, and theoretical). The degree of awareness of these issues and aims attributed to Freud is wide and divergent.

In this context, the present study falls into the category of those who take seriously Freud's explicit concern for truth. That is, it does not ascribe Freud some other agenda or latent conscious or unconscious motives (although such agendas and motives do seem to exist), but rather it underscores an understanding of the book that respects Freud's claim as to his own understanding of it. But, in contrast to other studies that take this concern seriously, it does not simply declare the book to be a failure, failing to offer an accurate or reasonable description of reality. This is not because the book is perceived as actually offering an accurate or reasonable description of reality, but rather because the intention to describe factual reality is but one major determinant of the nature of the book. Another is Freud's failure to do so. That is, it is the combination of the intention and failure that brings to the fore the special nature of the book. The present study suggests that *Moses and Monotheism* is at heart a depiction of a kind of reality, "historical truth," that cannot be captured by simple categories of true or false, fact or fantasy. And thus Freud's persistent return to his search for the fact of the matter, for material truth, despite all barriers, setbacks, and ongoing doubt, despite the unreasonableness of his method and findings, is precisely what expresses most forcefully the nature of this other kind of reality. It is in the way in which Freud fails to provide a reasonable account of actual history that he succeeds in sharing with his readers the meaning and nature of his encounter with historical truth, a truth that necessarily leads to such failure.

To highlight the distinction between this perspective and that which considers the value of the book in terms of its latent agendas, it should be noted that, from the present perspective, were Freud to gain greater self-awareness regarding the nature of his book, he would not have to recognize that he was offering fantasies, myths, psychodynamic speculations, creations of his mind or mistaken history, but rather that his own discoveries pertained to the realm of historical truth, not material truth, and that his methods for discovery and his categories for conceptualization were inadequate to deal with this realm. He would have to recognize that his attempt to describe the truth of Moses was partial, not because of his personal psychology or because his questions and concerns actually lay elsewhere, but rather because of limitations in his ability to describe the nature of the truth he was encountering. His insight here would in a sense be of a theoretical, not a psychological kind.

While Freud does, of course, specifically refer to historical truth, and the shifts to conviction despite doubt may reflect an implicit awareness of its manifestation in his own writing, this essential nature of the book seems to remain concealed from Freud himself.[6] It is perhaps because of the same limitations of our concepts and conceptual tendencies that subsequent reviewers have not sufficiently brought this dimension to the fore.

What allowed for this dimension to come to the fore in the present study points to another very significant aspect of the basic nature of Freud's *Moses* – its vitality and openness to the reader. It may be seen that in terms of forms or methods of investigation, in the present study I relied primarily on careful reading and analysis of Freud's texts, and awareness to the parallels between the content of Freud's writing and the process that he was undergoing in the course of writing. But in addition to these investigative methods, I felt that I was gaining a deeper understanding of Freud's intentions and ideas through their experiential revival within me. In the course of taking note of the puzzle that emerges in Freud's writing on Moses, in attempting to solve it through recognizing and gathering the fragments of which it is composed, and in bringing them together into a coherent whole, I felt that, strangely, I myself was taking part in many of the feelings that Freud was describing and experiencing in *Moses*. That is, as I began to deal with the puzzle, I felt a vague sense of certainty, at times a sure conviction, that the pieces of the puzzle that I was gathering were indeed the relevant ones, and that they somehow, in a way not yet known to me would indeed come together into a meaningful picture that would shed light on the issues at hand. I felt involved in a search for a truth that lies beyond the pieces, and that this search was guiding me along in moments of doubt. Ultimately, I could question the value of the coherence of the collected fragments, but could at the same time "know" that the desire for their coherence was here serving as a kind of impetus to a truth whose validity I could be sure of in some other, albeit not clearly defined, way. I gradually became aware that these kinds of experiential shifts that I was undergoing with varying degrees of intensity in the course of the preparation of the present chapter in a sense may have paralleled some of the shifts that Freud himself was undergoing in the course of the writing of *Moses* and were, in fact, opening me to a possible understanding of Freud's state of mind, and the reality that it reflected, in a very live way.

Freud's *Moses and Monotheism* can thus be understood not only as a book about conviction in a kind of truth that is not immediately amenable to simple demonstration, or as an expression of Freud's own enacted struggle with such truth, but also a book which allows the reader to join in and directly encounter this struggle. Beyond whatever literary techniques and pedagogic methods that Freud may have been actively employing in his *Moses* (Mahony, 1982), the book by its very nature allows the active reader, one coming with an enquiring stance and hope for discovery of truth regarding the depths of the human psyche, to reexperience through the study of the text the kinds of questions and feelings that tend to accompany such a quest for truth. It is through this active kind of reading that Freud's writings come alive and find their contemporary relevance (Blass, 2001). In my attempt to find the truth behind the puzzle of Freud's puzzle analogy they came alive for me, and allowed me a new understanding of Freud and more importantly, of the nature of the experience of truth that he too was seeking.

Notes

1 I refer here only to those instances in which Freud uses the term puzzle in the sense of a picture whose fragmented pieces are to be fitted together into a coherent whole. There are several additional senses in which he uses the term, but these are not relevant here.

2 To remain within the scope of the present chapter I put aside certain interesting differences between the 1896 and 1923 references that are to be found alongside the basic similarity.

3 This intermediate reality should not be confused with Winnicott's transitional space. For Freud this intermediate reality is created by a real external event, which then, in turn, shapes the mind and thus leaves the question of truth a real and relevant one, albeit not simply answered. In this sense Freud's notion is much closer to Laplanche's ideas regarding the "enigmatic message" (1995).

4 This experiential understanding finds support in Freud's more general attitude to dream interpretation as a source of relief (especially at the time when he was developing his ideas on doubt as lack of trust in love). In his 1908 introduction to his *Interpretation of Dreams* he writes that in working with the neuroses 'I have often been in doubt and sometimes been shaken in my convictions. At such times it has always been the *Interpretation of Dreams* [i.e. the book] that has given back my certainty. It is thus a sure instinct which has led my many scientific opponents to refuse to follow me more especially in my researches upon dreams' (p. xxvi).

5 In this chapter I have focused on this fear in the context of Freud's dream theory, but his fear of imposition in the context of his seduction theory, where Freud first introduces his puzzle analogy, should not be overlooked (Blass and Simon, 1992, 1994).

6 In this context, Freud's suggestion at one point that the subtitle of his book should be a *'historische Roman'* does not contradict the argument set forth here regarding this essential nature of the book, and may, in fact, further indicate some implicit awareness to it on Freud's part. In the introduction to the 1934 draft that includes this subtitle (in Yerushalmi, 1991, p. 17), Freud explicitly explains how in his use of the term *'historische Roman'* a new definition of the term is required that excludes the notions of fiction and invention ('associated with the blemish of error') that appear in common definitions of the term, but at the same time allows for a truth that has no proven reality. It should be added that this understanding of the nature of book in no way detracts from the claim that it has a day-dream-like quality (Grubrich-Simitis, 1997), but only offers an alternate explanation of the source of this quality. It is suggested that its source is in an encounter with a reality that Freud could not comprehend in the ways usually available to him.

References

Assmann, J. (1997). *Moses the Egyptian: The Memory of Egypt in Western Monotheism*. Cambridge, MA: Harvard Univ. Press.

Bernstein, R. J. (1998). *Freud and the Legacy of Moses*. Cambridge: Cambridge University Press.

Blass, R. B. (1992). Did Dora have an Oedipus? A re-examination of the theoretical context of Freud's 'Fragment of an analysis.' *Psychoanal. St. Child* 47: 159–187.

Blass, R. B. (2001). On the teaching of the Oedipus complex: On making Freud meaningful to university students by unveiling his essential ideas on the human condition. *Int. J. PsychoAnal.* 82: 1105–1121.
Blass, R. B. (2002). *The Meaning of the Dream in Psychoanalysis*. Albany: State University of New York Press.
Blass, R. B, & Simon, B. (1992). Freud on his own mistake(s): The role of seduction in the etiology of neurosis. *Psychiatry and the Humanities* 12: 160–183.
Blass, R. B. & Simon, B. (1994). The value of the historical perspective to contemporary psychoanalysis: Freud's seduction hypothesis. *Int. J. Psycho-Anal.* 75: 677–694.
Freud, E. (Ed.) (1960). *Letters of Sigmund Freud*. New York: Basic Books.
Freud, S. (1896). The Aetiology of Hysteria. *S.E.*3.
Freud, S. (1900). The Interpretation of Dreams. *S.E.*4.
Freud, S. (1909). Notes upon a Case of Obsessional Neurosis. *S.E.*10.
Freud, S. (1912–13). Totem and Taboo. *S.E.*13.
Freud, S (1915). The Dynamics of Transference. *S.E.*11.
Freud, S. (1923). Remarks on the Theory and Practice of Dream-Interpretation. *S.E.*19.
Freud, S. (1927). The Future of an Illusion. *S.E.*21.
Freud, S. (1935). Postscript to an Autobiographical Study. *S.E.* 20.
Freud, S. (1939). Moses and Monotheism. *S.E.*23.
Grubrich-SimitisI (1997). *Early Freud and Late Freud: Reading Anew Studies on Hysteria and Moses and Monotheism*. London: Routledge.
Laplanche, J. (1995). Seduction, persecution, revelation. *Int. J. Psycho-Anal.* 76: 663–682.
Mahony, P. (1982). *Freud as a Writer*. New York: Int. Univ. Press.
Meissner, W. (1971). Freud's methodology. *J. Amer. Psychoanal. Assn.* 19: 265–309.
Paul, R. (1994). Freud, Sellin and the death of Moses. *Int. J. Psycho-Anal.* 75: 825–837.
Paul, R. (1996). *Moses and Civilization: The Meaning behind Freud's Myth*. New Haven: Yale Univ. Press.
Pfeiffer, E. (ed.) (1966). *Sigmund Freud and Lou Andreas-Salomé: Letters*. New York: Harcourt, Brace, Jovanovich.
Rice, E. (1990). *Freud and Moses: The Long Journey Home*. Albany: State Univ. of New York Press.
Rogers, R. (1981). Textuality in dreams. *Int. Rev. Psycho-Anal.* 8: 433–447.
Spence, D. (1982). Narrative truth and theoretical truth. *Psychoanal. Q.* 51: 43–69.
Steele, R. (1979). Psychoanalysis and hermeneutics. *Int. Rev. Psycho-Anal.* 6: 389–411.
Yerushalmi, Y. H. (1991). *Freud's Moses: Judaism Terminable and Interminable*. New Haven: Yale Univ. Press.

Editor's Introduction to Chapter 8

Lawrence J. Brown

Shmuel Erlich examines Freud's complicated relationship to Judaism within the context of *leadership*: Moses' stewardship of the Israelites as he guided them out of bondage and into the Promised Land and Freud's leadership of the psychoanalytic movement. *Moses and Monotheism* is for Erlich a "multifaceted and strange work" (this volume) that has been discussed from many perspectives, but his emphasis in this chapter is on Moses and Freud as leaders. Erlich writes that

> Freud is deeply concerned with Moses the leader of men, and his concern grows directly out of his own identity and his leadership position.
>
> (Ibid.)

For Erlich, Moses' great accomplishment as a leader is to have transformed the newly liberated Semitic tribes into the Jewish people who are held together by their unconscious connection to their leader, Moses. Erlich applies Freud's (1921) theories about group formation to explain the complex processes by which the group coheres: the Leader (Moses) is experienced by the group members as an ego ideal with whom the Followers identify. Thus, the group is formed around a shared identification with the Leader's ego ideal.

Erlich also introduces us to Freud's notion of The Great Man:

> How is it possible for a single man to evolve such extraordinary effectiveness that he can form a people out of random individuals and families, can stamp them with their definitive character and determine their fate for thousands of years?
>
> (Freud, 1939, p. 107)

In this regard, Freud and Moses are both Great Men, each of whom are equally venerated and feared, and are determined to see their contributions – psychoanalysis and the Jewish people – continue to thrive and nourish their respective groups into the future. However, Erlich warns us that there are destructive processes in groups that work to undermine

DOI: 10.4324/9781003272045-16

their valued creations. Just as Akhenaten's heretical innovations were ultimately undone by revanchist forces in Egyptian society, so Freud's "heresies" had to be protected from the impact of his theories on society, and Moses ultimately was brought down by the people he led and by whom he was to be murdered (according to Freud).

Erlich also discusses the dynamics of anti-Semitism, describing two kinds: "ordinary" anti-Semitism which is rooted in the *neurotic* ambivalence of admiration for, and hatred of, Jews. Nazism, in contrast, is a *perverse psychotic* organization that seeks to annihilate anything and anyone whose being is at odds with the murderous precepts of the Third Reich. With regard to the spread of Nazism, Erlich keenly observes that Hitler's rise to power followed on Freud's (1921) observations about leadership in the group in which "his skillful and successful substitution of himself as the ego-ideal of an entire nation and large portions of humanity" (Erlich, this volume).

Paradoxically, Hitler may also be seen as a 'Great Man,' but as a dark inverse shadow, a vampire sucking the life out of mankind's triumphs.

The author (LJB) thanks Dr. Shmuel Erlich for giving permission to reprint his 2019 paper, Der Mann Moses and the Man Freud: Leadership, Legacy and Anti-Semitism. In *The Couch in the Marketplace: Psychoanalysis and Social Reality*, pp. 145–161.

8 Der Mann Moses and the Man Freud

Leadership, Legacy, and Anti-Semitism

Shmuel Erlich

"Freud is dead." This simple exclamatory statement opens Ernst Jones' obituary of Sigmund Freud. In his 25-page essay, in which he admirably summarizes Freud's personality and achievements, there is but one brief allusion to Freud's Jewishness. Referring to the "man Freud," it essentially recapitulates Freud's own acknowledgement (which I shall allude to later) with one small addition that has the slightest anti-Semitic trace:

> One cannot describe *the man Freud* without laying stress on the fact that he was a Jew. Though never orthodox or in any way religious he held together with his people, was a Governor of the Hebrew University in Jerusalem, and took an interest in all that concerned the fate of Jewry. The Nazi intolerance of this spared him no more than it had Einstein. The fact itself is of more than personal interest, since it is doubtful if without certain traits inherited from his Jewish ancestry Freud would have been able to accomplish the work he did. I think here of *a peculiar native shrewdness*, a skeptical attitude towards illusion and deception, and a determined courage that made him impervious to hostile public opinion and the contumely of his professional colleagues.
>
> (Jones, 1940; my emphasis)

Sigmund Freud's Jewishness was indeed never questionable. His anti-religious stance, his doubts and fears concerning the Zionist movement and its political feasibility, and his determined strivings toward scientific universalism – all of these could not mask or eradicate the deeply rooted and essential Jewish core of his identity. In the preface that he contributed to the Hebrew edition of *Totem and Taboo*, he stated this clearly:

> No reader of [the Hebrew version of] this book will find it easy to put himself in the emotional position of an author who is ignorant of the language of holy writ, who is completely estranged from the religion of his fathers – as well as from every other religion – and who cannot take a share in nationalist ideas, but who has yet never repudiated his people, who feels that he is in his essential nature a Jew and who has

DOI: 10.4324/9781003272045-17

> no desire to alter that nature. If the question were put to him: "Since you have abandoned all these common characteristics of your countrymen, what is there left to you that is Jewish?" he would reply: "A very great deal, and probably its very essence." He could not now express that essence clearly in words; but *some day, no doubt, it will become accessible to the scientific mind.*
>
> (1913, p. xv, my emphasis)

That day came during the period of 1934 to 1938, in which Freud wrote his *Man Moses* and, after much hesitation and soul-searching finally published it, immediately after his forced escape from Vienna that so willingly surrendered to Nazism. The work is unique among Freud's writings for many reasons. I would like to examine the closely intertwined links between Freud's dilemma with his Jewish identity, his deep concerns about his leadership and the future of his legacy, and his understanding of the position of the Jews in the world in relation to anti-Semitism. All these factors have important implications for the psychoanalytic identity as well as for the understanding of anti-Semitism.

Let me explain why I chose to call this essay "*Der Mann Moses*, the Man Freud." Of the numerous ways in which this multifaceted and strange work has been read, I am not so much drawn to its anti-religious, bible-critical, natural historical, literary-romantic, and even Jewish-nationalistic aspects. All of these and more have been dealt with quite extensively. What captivates my imagination is the title Freud gave this work: "*Der Mann Moses und die Monoteistische Religion*" [literally translated: The Man Moses and the Monotheistic Religion]. My emphasis falls on "*Der Mann Moses*" and its obvious parallel: "*The man Freud.*"

"The Man Moses" is actually a biblical phrase, and it is reasonable to assume that Freud was familiar with it. If we look for its source, we find it mentioned only twice, both times in Exodus and in the context of Moses' leadership. The first time has a distinctly positive color:

> And the Lord gave the people favour in the sight of the Egyptians. Moreover, the man Moses was very great in the land of Egypt, in the sight of Pharaoh's servants, and in the sight of the people.
>
> (Exodus 11:3)

The second occurrence is in the context of the sin of the creation of the Golden Calf, and has a decidedly negative cast:

> And when the people saw that Moses delayed to come down from the mount, the people gathered themselves together unto Aaron, and said to him: "Up, make us a god who shall go before us; for as for this Moses, the man that brought us out of the land of Egypt, we know not what is become of him."
>
> (Exodus 32:1)

The negative connotation is further emphasized by the reversal of the order: Rather than "the man Moses" it is now "Moses the man," i.e., Moses who is after all only a man and not a god. The appearance of the phrase "The Man Moses" in the context of *leadership* is significant to the line of thought I wish to develop.

The Man Moses occupies a special niche in the corpus of Freud's writings. The continuing fascination with this singular work is probably due to the many dynamic strands woven into it. The author's semi-awareness of personal allusions and connections lends it an air of a self-reflective look at a long and productive life. It might well be the last stage in Freud's life-long self-analysis, which began with and consisted largely in the analysis of his dreams. *Moses and Monotheism* might be viewed as a dream dreamt late in Freud's life and its interpretation. Perhaps this is implied in the subtitle of this work, "*Ein Historischer Roman*" [A Historic Novel or Fiction], a subtitle that "inevitably …conjures up associations to both fiction and the psychoanalytic 'family romance' (*Familienroman*)" (Yerushalmi, 1989).Seen this way, its thematic richness immediately beckons to our imagination.

To mention a few of these themes: It is Freud's last and most telling attack on Jewish narcissism. It aims to resolve once and for all the riddle of the internal and external "specialness" of the Jews. The Chosen (and therefore persecuted) People is transformed into the tragically Guilty People, forever atoning for their crime, but at the same time internalizing and transforming carnage and murder into spirituality and valued cultural possessions for all mankind. Above all, however, it is Freud's most daring foray into the area of spirituality, or *Geistigkeit*. It must be pointed out (as already remarked by Strachey, the editor of the Standard Edition of Freud's writings) that *Geistigkeit*, a word which I will make use of repeatedly in what follows, is hardly translatable into English. It combines the related but not at all synonymous meanings of mind, spirit, and intellect, as well as a hint at loftiness and transcendence. Strachey's choice to translate it mostly as "intellectuality," probably to avoid its metaphysical connotations, does not do it justice, and was likely guided by consideration for Freud's usual aversion of such connotations.

We must bear in mind that Freud embraced Helmholtzian empiricism and had forsworn all metaphysical efforts. His life's work was to transform "spirit" and "soul" into the relatively more empirical "mind" and "mental apparatus," and divine inspiration into the ultimately somatically and biologically derived Unconscious. He is also the man who confessed, in response to Romain Rolland's assertion of the existence of "oceanic" feelings, that he "cannot discover this 'oceanic' feeling in [him] self" (Freud, 1930, p. 65). For him to delve into the issue of *Geistigkeit* was certainly significant.

Freud's effort to understand *Geistigkeit* has to do with yet another struggle: his attempt to integrate his parochial Jewish identity with his allegiance to the prevailing non-Jewish, largely anti-Semitic, Central European culture through scientific universalism. In this pursuit Freud is, of course, an outstanding example of the heroic efforts of Jewish Enlightenment, from Moses Mendelssohn (another Moses!) onward, to reconcile Jewish separatism with the prevailing Christian culture. Freud's efforts to save psychoanalysis from becoming "a Jewish science" led to his anointment of C. G. Jung as his heir and future leader of the psychoanalytic movement. Jung was to be his Joshua (the identification with Moses is again pivotal) – an Aryan, powerful conqueror of the new land. That this attempt failed miserably is well known; it is also painfully implicit in Freud's *Moses*: a last attempt to unravel, and at the same time to accept, the riddle of Jewish isolationism, the split between Judaism and Christianity, or better yet: between being Jewish and being Gentile – the two that were one and became inseparable antagonists.

Another aspect of the special attractiveness of this work is its prophetic quality in terms of historical timing and cultural significance. The struggle between Jewishness and Worldliness, whether of Christian or neo-pagan cast, was about to erupt full force in the form of Nazi ideology and persecution. Freud's initial hesitation and eventual decision to publish this work following his escape to England (his "exile" to a new Diaspora) are poignant themes that operate powerfully in the background. The tremendous attraction and fascination of Freud's *Moses* owes much to this uncanny intertwining of the personal with the historical, of the intellectual analysis with the actual experience and fate of the Man Freud.

As I said, I will not expand on these fascinating issues. I would like to take up a theme, which though implicit in what was already mentioned, to the best of my knowledge has not been described and discussed as such. This theme touches on the deep connection between the Man Freud and *Der Mann Moses*. It is the theme of *leadership*. In turn, it is also closely related to *identity*, as well as to anti-Semitism and Freud's understanding of it.

Briefly stated, my thesis is this: Freud is deeply concerned with Moses the leader of men, and his concern grows directly out of his own identity and his leadership position. The "socio-historical" analysis of the Man Moses is indeed self-serving, and represents a complex and deep identification: it strives to enlighten the Man Freud about the fate and future of his own leadership. Moreover, this perspective is intrinsically associated with the historical and social role of the Jews and the hatred directed at them in the form of anti-Semitism.

Freud the Leader

That Freud's identity contained a major leadership component is undisputable. His interest in and early identification with Hannibal and Alexander the Great, with ancient and contemporary political leaders and military heroes is well known (Jones, 1953; Gay, 1988). A variant of this quest for leadership took the form of identifying with the great discoverers and a passion to achieve fame through scientific discoveries. Forging ahead, establishing and seizing new uncharted territories, claiming and civilizing the unknown and uninitiated – these themes are evident in much of his thinking and writing. It takes the form of bringing the light of truth, insight, and enlightenment to the "heathens," the unaware and uninformed.

From this perspective, Freud is actually no less concerned with the figure of Paul than with Moses. Paul is responsible for the transformation of Judaism into Christianity, by offering the pagan world a way out from patricidal guilt. Both men (Paul and Moses) are Jews; both transformed mankind and left their indelible mark on it. Freud's preferential focus, however, is clearly on Moses and not on Paul. I believe this is in part because Moses is the earlier and more original figure, but even more so because he is credited with the miraculous transformation of the nomadic Semitic tribes into the Jewish people. In this sense Moses represents much better the profound potential and far-reaching effects of leadership. Moreover, Moses is directly connected with the roots of anti-Semitism, whereas Paul represents its possible resolution by negating and abandoning the Jewish identity, a solution historically rejected by the Jews as much as by Freud himself. The conflict represented by Moses and Paul is the issue out of which anti-Semitism springs onto the scene of history. It is therefore significant that Freud clearly chooses Moses over Paul, confirming once again his Jewish identity, while also recognizing and even mourning the tragic and inevitable consequences of his choice.

Freud on Leadership

Before I let Freud speak for himself on this score, his thoughts about group process and leadership must be briefly reviewed. Freud made numerable forays into cultural and social areas, culminating in his *Moses*. They represent the application of psychoanalytic principles and concepts, forged in the arena of the individual psyche and dyadic setting, to the supra-individual level. In effect, Freud pursued an approach I have described as "summation" (Erlich, 1996) in his understanding of group and social phenomena. In this approach, the processes that occur in the group (the horde or the mass) are derived directly from the individual psyche, and are then summed up across numerous participants. The group, in this conception, is not really a new or emergent phenomenon, obeying its own dynamics, but the sum of the individual psyches within it. To underscore this additive approach (which is not only Freud's), one may contrast it with the next development in the psychoanalytic understanding of group processes, which is associated with Bion (1961). Unlike Freud, Bion views the group as possessing characteristics that transcend the individual member's psychic processes. Employing post-Freudian Kleinian concepts, Bion arrives at a "group-as-a-whole" dimension, expressed in his notions of a proto-mental level and Basic Assumption groups. These operate covertly at the group level, and usurp individuals to their own ends.

Freud's groundbreaking effort at understanding group processes, his *Group Psychology and the Analysis of the Ego* (1921), is the first attempt to construct a psychoanalytic explanation of group processes. While basically following the scheme I just described – i.e., summation of individual psychic processes as the explanation for what transpires in groups – it is nevertheless striking in terms of its conceptual analysis and focus, which is clearly on *leadership*. Freud divides the group into two major components: Leader and Followers. What makes a group cohere is the group members' replacement of their individual ego-ideal with that of the leader. The leader thus becomes invested as the common ego-ideal (or ideal self) that the group is willing and ready to follow. It is as if the leader's ego-ideal has occupied the place previously held by the personal ego-ideal in each follower's mind, so that each follower now measures himself and fashions his aspirations in the image of the internalized leader. In addition, group members identify with each other in their common idealization of the leader.

Two elements in Freud's *Group Psychology* are noteworthy here, and both are intrinsically related to his preoccupation with *The Man Moses*. In the first place, Freud attributes the moment of *group formation*, as well as its continued existence, to the presence of *leadership*. Without the advent of the leader the group would not come into being and the social process would grind to a halt. Freud draws on the primal horde as the primitive constituent of the group: "The leader of the group is still the dreaded primal father; the group still wishes to be governed by unrestricted force; it has *an extreme passion for authority*; …it has a thirst for obedience" (1921, p. 127, my emphasis). Freud's view of authority is clearly vertical, and derives from a child's relatedness to his father: authority comes from above, and is yearned for from below. He seems to have no notion at all of the possibility of horizontal authorization – of being authorized by one's peers.

The second observation follows directly from the first: The process by which the group is formed is from the top down. Employing the primal horde metaphor, it is literally created and held together by the action of the primal, ruthless father. This notion is related to Hegelian dialectics of leader and follower, or master and slave. In the structural analysis of psychoanalyst-anthropologist Robert Paul (1996), Freud's *Moses* deals with the relationship between a senior-dominant male and junior-submissive males.

I wish to underscore Freud's immense valuation, perhaps even overvaluation, of the leader's role in the inception and structuring of the process of group formation and group action. The dynamics are analogous to loving, as in suggestion and hypnosis, though he certainly notes the presence of fear as well. The investiture of the leader is essentially a narcissistic act, as the ego-ideal is invested with narcissistic libido. The leader is the one loved by all (with the caveat that this love is ambivalent). Moreover, he is the one that everyone wishes to be equally loved by. The obliteration of differences and the acceptance of sameness (equality?) by group members are attributed to their identification with each other in their common love for the leader. What Freud does not fully take into account, precisely for the same reason that prevents him from appreciating the "oceanic" feeling, is the fusion and merger-like nature of narcissistic love. Indeed, the love and idealized aspirations of the followers toward the leader imply a powerful wish to merge and become one with him. In other words, there is a dynamic propulsion toward *obliterating* one's singular, bounded self, by merging it with the potentially offered, overarching unity and oneness of the group. Such merger tendencies operate especially powerfully in large groups, but are also present in small groups, and to an extent even in work groups (Erlich, 1996, 2000). The merger experience represents the potential promise of regaining the self after losing it in the group in a form and state that are not merely superior, but more importantly – are essential for assuming an identity. *Identity formation* is contingent not only on being able to establish self-definition, but also upon one's capacity to merge and feel at-one with a given social role and the community that offers it. I will come back to this point, since it relates to anti-Semitism in general and to the Nazi phenomenon in particular.

For Freud, the leader is unquestionably The Great Man, with an obvious allusion to the *physically* Big Man (*Der Grosse Mann*) or Father, whose psychic place and aura he assumes, together with the father's authority, approval and precious love. The question that preoccupies Freud throughout *Moses* is the one he explicitly poses about this Great Man: "How is it possible for a single man to evolve such extraordinary effectiveness that he can form a people out of random individuals and families, can stamp them with their definitive character and determine their fate for thousands of years?" (1939, p. 107). That this question sends him back in time and represents a deep personal puzzlement, touching the foundations of his earliest development and identity formation, is suggested by the immediately following sentence:

> Is not a hypothesis such as this *a relapse* into the mode of thought which led to myths of a creator and to the worship of heroes, into times in which the writing of history was nothing more than a report of the deeds and destinies of single individuals, of rulers or conquerors?
>
> (ibid., my emphasis)

Freud is well aware that modern scientific thinking has a clear preference for impersonal forces, in which "individuals have no other part to play… than as exponents or representatives of group trends" (ibid.). This remark, incidentally, anticipates the Open Systems theory discussed above (Chapter 2). Nonetheless, he insists upon the place of the Great Man in the chain or network of causes. Difficult as it may be to define this greatness, he asserts that we should "take it for granted that a great man influences his fellow men in two ways: by his personality and *by the idea which he puts forward*" (ibid., p. 109, my emphasis). (Perhaps not coincidentally, these are also the attributes that Jones refers to in his obituary [1940].) And Freud adds pointedly:

> Not for a moment are we in the dark as to why a great man ever becomes important. We know that in the mass of mankind there is a powerful need for an authority which can be admired, before whom one bows down, by whom one is ruled and perhaps even ill-treated... It is a longing for the father felt by everyone from his childhood onwards ... The decisiveness of thought, the strength of will, the energy of action are part of the picture of a father – but above all the autonomy and independence of the great man, his divine unconcern which may grow into ruthlessness. One must admire him, one may trust him, but one cannot avoid being afraid of him too.
>
> (Ibid., pp. 109–110)

Moses is the man who assumed this paternal role of the great man, offering "the poor Jewish bondsmen" an object for their devotion: a God whom they could worship and obey in return for his love, and whose wrath and punishment they could fear. The tradeoff is between being the Chosen Children of God in return for paying eternal allegiance to him.

All of this is over-determined and heavily suffused with personal meaning. The identities of the two Great Men – Moses and Freud – have become intertwined, with the Jewish people actively cementing their fusion. Let us note, as Erikson (1968) already did, that the only time Freud used the word "*identity*" in his formidable corpus of writing is when he alluded to his *Jewish* identity. In his letter to the B'nai B'rith Society on his seventieth birthday he said:

> Plenty of other things remained over to make the attraction of Jewry and Jews irresistible – many obscure emotional forces, which were the more powerful the less they could be expressed in words, as well as a clear consciousness of *inner identity*... It was to my Jewish nature alone that I owed two characteristics that had become indispensable to me in the difficult course of my life. Because I was a Jew I found myself free from many prejudices which restricted others in the use of their intellect; and as a Jew I was prepared to join the Opposition and to do without agreement with the "compact majority"...
>
> *At a time when no one in Europe listened to me and I still had no disciples* even in Vienna, you gave me your kindly attention. You were my first audience.
>
> (1926, pp. 273–274, my emphasis)

Freud's words disclose striking connections between these deeply personal themes: his inner identity is closely linked with being a Jew *and* with being a leader. The latter is clearly expressed in a number of ways: his capacity and readiness for taking up non-consensual positions, and his long frustrated but persistent need for followership. Both these themes are intriguingly intertwined with the Man Moses and inform his *Moses*. Let me elaborate.

Leadership can be defined in many ways. I have already mentioned Freud's attempt to account for the Great Man phenomenon. The more current conception of leadership, to which I subscribe, is based upon the integration of psychoanalytic concepts and understanding, based largely on the work of Melanie Klein and Bion, with the structural and systemic view of organizational life offered by Open System theory. This unique integration (discussed above in Chapter 2) contributed much to a deeper understanding of group processes. Within this frame, leadership is seen as a boundary phenomenon: "Leadership of the group, like that of the individual, is a *boundary function* that controls transactions between inside and outside" (Miller & Rice, 1967, p. 20, my emphasis). It is the leader's willingness to take up this position, which is also fraught with considerable danger, which makes him a leader.[1]

Freud's own aspirations and personal readiness to take up such a boundary position is clearly reflected in the above quoted passage as well as in numerous other ways. He is always ready to forgo "the compact majority" in which he might comfortably lose himself. To be sure, to be in the opposition, in and of itself, is not yet to take up a leadership role. The opposition is, however, a way of drawing a line of disagreement or boundary. In this instance, the new boundary drawn is psychoanalysis, and it is Freud himself who draws it. He is therefore not merely *in* the opposition; he *is* the opposition. He draws this boundary and takes up his position on it for his entire adult life. This clearly puts him in a leadership role and position. That he is only too painfully aware of it is reflected in his woeful statement about the absence of disciples and followers for such a long time.

But Freud is not alone in this boundary stance: the Jewish people, as he sees it, are in a leadership role vis-à-vis the rest of the world. This, of course, is not a novel idea. It is the essence of Jewish tradition, which Freud must have taken in from early on. What is significant is how fully he has adopted it, though not entirely without ambivalence and difficulty. His own leadership has become identified with Jewish spiritual leadership. This is where Moses enters the scene. Moses holds the key to the riddle with which Freud, the latter day solver of the riddle of the Sphinx, but also the Giver of the Law of dreams and the Unconscious, is grappling. It is the riddle presented by old age, imminent death and the issue of legacy and transmission. Having been so immensely generative, he is now concerned with *continuity* – with the durability and permanence of his achievements. The question for Freud, at this point in his life, is not the survival of the Jews or his own personal safety. What is at stake, as it has been at a number of previous junctures in the course of his leadership, is the survival of psychoanalysis *as he conceived it*. From a contemporary perspective, only some seventy years later, it sometimes looks as if indeed he had good cause for concern.

Moses is almost interchangeable with Freud in this regard. He too is depicted as a person who does not need the compact majority, which in his case consists of the priests who oppose Pharaoh Akhenaton's reforms. He is a man of single-minded dedication to an idea that runs counter to the prevailing cultural beliefs, social norms, and personal experience. His abstract conception of an imageless, non-corporeal God is the boundary he creates, setting him off from the rest of mankind. He is therefore the everlasting proof that an *idea* can be so tremendously transformative as to sweep and forever change an entire people and culture. Moses signifies that spirituality and ideology can win the day and forever change the course of history.

This is precisely the proof that Freud is seeking at this point in his life. Having almost single-handedly placed psychoanalysis on the cultural stage of the twentieth century, he needs to know that his ideas and spiritual force will survive and continue to exist after him. His question is addressed to himself as much as to his followers and successors: Will they forever adhere to his teachings? Will his legacy be stamped in them for all times, as the Jews have internalized Moses and his teachings? Will these teachings and ideas withstand the test of time, and yet be capable of adapting to changing circumstances?

Moses provides a source of hope and a positive horizon for this dilemma. At the same time, however, Freud is also aware of the tragic dimension involved. The leader's position on the boundary makes him the target and object of the group's aggression. Placing oneself on the boundary is an act of courage, precisely because one may be abruptly transformed into *The Enemy* of the group (Erlich, 1997). Yet Freud's tragic insight into this dilemma goes deeper still: the lesson he draws from his reconstruction of Moses is that for the leader's legacy to be internalized, *he must first be killed by the group*. Spiritual elevation and ideological internalization hinge upon the destructive devouring of the person who stands for and symbolizes these (Freud, 1913). Murder, cannibalistic incorporation, and totemic worship thus serve as the fulcrum for the spiritual, mental, and intellectual advances of *Geistigkeit*. The lofty spiritual heights of which man is capable cannot be regarded merely as the refined, sublimated, and acculturated derivatives of instinctual drives, unrecognizably transformed. They must be re-possessed again and again through transformational and incorporative processes that are drive-propelled. Ideas are taken in and assimilated through the murderous annihilation of those who represent them. The internalization of the *Geistig* occurs through the aggressive obliteration of the leader who represents it.

We may wish to debate Freud's inherently pessimistic view of the advancement of human spirituality. Personally, I think there is much to it. One particular aspect of Freud's legacy is especially worthy of contemplation: spiritual and ideological matters are certainly not the pristine, otherworldly, non-pragmatic and realistically equivocal factors they often are depicted to be in a commercial and power-oriented world. *No aggression is remotely comparable to the aggression generated by an idea.* This should not, and cannot, be dismissed as mere irrationality, to be overcome by rationality and pragmatism. Ideas and ideologies engender so much aggression because of the need to destroy their carriers, in order to defend the *purity* of one's own beliefs. Freud's *Moses* suggests that such aggression is but the first step toward the incorporation of such menacing new ideas. The destructiveness is often projected *outwardly* onto others-enemies who must be annihilated in the name of the purity demanded by one's own ideals. Some of this aggression is channeled back into the group, where it is expressed in ideological struggles and factionalism.

The Roots of Anti-Semitism

Living in Jerusalem provides ample evidence of the destructive power of ideologies and of the death wishes that ideas are capable of evoking. Similar difficulties plague most of the world today. The issue of Jewish identity, about which so much has been said and written, is rooted in the eternal dilemma that Moses bequeathed to the Jews: Are they to be a people like all others, or must they forever follow a special task and destiny? To choose the second option means to live constantly on the boundary: that is, to take up a *leadership* position vis-à-vis the rest of the world, with the attendant hatred, aggression, and persecution, as well as admiration and fascination, this position evokes and attracts. History shows that even when the Jews preferred to be like all others and to repudiate this leadership role, the others were not likely to accept this lightly. It seems to support and provide evidence for Freud's thesis that the roots of anti-Semitism are in the sphere of *Geistigkeit*, in being the willing or unwilling representative of the *Geistig*, or the spiritual, for the rest of mankind. The world cannot fully reject the *Geistig* because without it, it will not be truly human. But it can hate, despise and express its ambivalence by hating, despising, rejecting, and persecuting those who stand for it.

The course of human evolution, as captured by Darwin and Freud, and supported by modern genetic science, runs an uninterrupted course from the inanimate to the animalistic to the spiritual. Freud (1920) had already focused on the transition from inanimate matter to life forms. The Life and Death drives are the forces that capture this moment of transition, conserving and preserving the dynamic swing to life, as well as its undoing. In the *Man Moses*, he focuses on *the transition from animism and paganism to abstract faith, and from concrete animism to the dominance of the spiritual and the intellectual.* This is the crucial shift that enables the mind to imagine and to think, to go beyond perceptual impressions and sense presentations to mental representations, to symbolism and abstraction. Bion (1962) refers to this transformational capability as the *alpha function*. It is perhaps the single most important developmental step mankind has taken, breaking loose of the stranglehold of the senses and their sense-presentations. Just like freeing ourselves of the gravitational pull of the Earth requires enormous energy and explosive force, setting the mind free similarly depends on explosive energy. This energy derives from Man's capacity to hate and destroy, but also to love and mourn, as in Freud's fictitious reconstruction of the murder of Moses. The explosion set off by that murder, the explosion that created the Jewish people, has never subsided. Like a volcano, its ripples continue to rumble underneath the surface, erupting with horrendous irrationality and directing enormous energies of hatred and destruction against the surviving witnesses of the original explosion. The struggle that created *Geistigkeit* continues to erupt in the form of the hatred of the Jews.

Anti-Semitism, as Freud clearly understood, is therefore forever intertwined with the story of mankind. It partakes of the ambivalence and hatred we feel toward our parents for giving us life and for being there before us, and even more so – for representing morality and the strictures and constraints imposed upon our instinctual freedom. The neurotic individual ambivalently submits to these parental prohibitions and internalizes them. He idealizes his parents, at the same time that he suffers from the hate and aggression he unconsciously directs at them and their substitutes. The perverse individual, on the other hand, never accepts or internalizes these feelings, and is endlessly engaged in a destructive process of iconoclastic deconstruction – in an attempt to destroy their signifiers, concretely and/or symbolically. The perverse *wish* is to create a world free from the burdens of parents, morality, and spirituality, from historical and interpersonal diversity and generational differences. As a result, the perverse individual lives in an empty and desolate world in which his loneliness and emptiness are only momentarily relieved by manic defenses of "action" and "doing." A perverse society is similarly doomed to self-destruction and the annihilation of its future. Nazi ideology represents precisely such a perverse solution.

There is a deep chasm between "ordinary" anti-Semitism and Nazism. Anti-Semitism rests on neurotic ambivalence, in which love and admiration for the Jews conflict with hatred for everything they symbolize. Nazism, on the other hand, represents the perverse *wish and its enactment* – as in all perversions – to create a new world, free of Jews and the *Geistigkeit* they represent. Nazi ideology expresses the perverse psychotic wish to obliterate differentiated civilization, painstakingly built upon the recognition of differences – between men and women, between generations, between different families and societies – and the respect accorded to these differences under the Law. The prevailing traditional European anti-Semitism provided the fertile soil and momentum for this psychotic wish to take hold, to overtake and sweep the entire German society and culture in its wake (Bursztein, 1998 [2004]). Hitler's assumption of leadership occurred precisely through the dynamics that Freud had keenly foreseen and described: his skillful and successful substitution of himself as the ego-ideal of an entire nation and large portions of humanity.

The risk of my discussion so far is that it might lead to the conclusion that anti-Semitism, especially in its perverse Nazi form, is a mere historical phenomenon and a thing of the past. Such a conclusion would indeed be a dangerously misleading illusion. Anti-Semitism is alive and well, currently taking refuge under the new guise of anti-Israel sentiments and hatred. Since my vantage point in this discussion is psychoanalytic and social, rather than political, I will not dwell on this theme. Instead I will quote from a recent interview with a Hebrew University of Jerusalem historian, in which he asserts that:

- Not since 1945 has there been such a level of concern, anxiety, or depression among Europe's Jews as one witnesses today. The newly emerging Europe is turning out to be the worst of all possible worlds for its Jews.
- Anti-Semitism is a primary symptom of Europe's pathology. Every society that becomes seriously infected by it is receiving a wakeup call about its social, cultural, and political health.
- Often the same Europeans who oppose the more obvious, uncontroversial manifestations of anti-Semitism encourage it – wittingly or unwittingly – through their overall posture on Israel (Wistrich, 2004).

An additional form that current anti-Semitism takes is the denial of the Holocaust. A relevant illustration of this can be found in the trial judgment of British historian David Irvin.[2]

The struggle between spirituality and the enlightened intellect on one hand, and the hatred for those who signify it, is far from over. Anti-Semitism, in my view, can erupt in places and cultures that have never even seen a Jew. Because it stems from the struggle between the drives and *Geistigkeit*, it will always be present in one form or another. It will usually be directed against those who symbolize the momentous transition in which spirituality, consciousness, and rationality emerged and were chosen over instinctual satisfaction. This is the legacy of Freud's psychoanalysis, of his *Man Moses* and of the Jews, whoever they may be at a given moment in the history of mankind.

Notes

1 It is striking that Freud was aware of and made use of this boundary notion. Two of his main concepts involve being on the boundary: Instinctual drive (*Trieb*), responsible for so much initiative and wishful action, is "on the frontier between the mental and the somatic" (1915, p. 122). And the ego (*das Ich*), the subsystem of the mind that provides internal leadership, functions as a "frontier-creature, ...[that] tries to mediate between the world and the id" (1923, p. 56). This is consistent with sophisticated current organizational thinking.

2 See www.hdot.org/trial/judgement

References

Bion, W. R. (1961) *Experiences in Groups*. London: Tavistock Publications.

Bursztein, J.-G. (1998) *Hitler, la tyrannie et la psychoanalyse: Essai sur la destruction de la civilization*. Nouvelles Etudes Freudiennes. [Hebrew Edition: Tel Aviv: Resling Publishing, 2004].

Erikson, E. H. (1968) *Identity, Youth and Crisis*. New York: Norton.

Erlich, H. S. (1996) Ego and self in the group. *Group Analysis*, 29: 229–243.

Erlich, H. S. (1997) On discourse with an enemy. In: Edward R. Shapiro (Ed.), *The Inner World in the Outer World: Psychoanalytic Perspectives*. New Haven: Yale University Press, pp. 123–142.

Erlich, H. S. (2000) Joining, experiencing, and individuating: Ego and self in the group. In Bruna Seu (Ed.), *Who Am I? The Ego and the Self in Psychoanalysis*. London: Rebus Press, pp. 128–142.

Freud, S. (1913) Totem and Taboo. *S.E.*, 13: 1–161.

Freud, S. (1915) Instincts and Their Vicissitudes. *S.E.*, 14: 117–140.

Freud, S. (1920) Beyond the Pleasure Principle. *S.E.*, 18: 7–64.

Freud, S. (1921) Group Psychology and the Analysis of the Ego. *S.E.*, 18: 69–143.

Freud, S. (1923) The Ego and the Id. *S.E.*, 19: 1–59.

Freud, S. (1926) Address to the Society of B'nai B'rith. *S.E.*, 20: 273–274.

Freud, S. (1930) Civilization and Its Discontents. *S.E.*, 21: 64–145.

Freud, S. (1939) Moses and Monotheism: Three Essays. *S.E.*, 23: 7–137.

Gay, P. (1988) *Freud: A Life for Our Time*. New York: Norton.

Jones, E. (1940) Sigmund Freud 1856–1939. *Int. J. Psycho-Anal.*, 21: 2–26.

Jones, E. (1953) *The Life and Work of Sigmund Freud*. Vol. 1 (1856–1900). New York: Basic Books.

Miller, E. J. and Rice, A. K. (1967) *Systems of Organization*. London: Tavistock Publications.

Paul, R. A. (1996) *Moses and Civilization: The Meaning behind Freud's Myth*. New Haven: Yale University Press.

Wistrich, R. (2004) *Post-Holocaust and Anti-Semitism*, No. 25, October 1, 2004.

Yerushalmi, Y. (1989) Freud on the 'Historical Novel': From the manuscript draft (1934) of Moses and Monotheism. *Int. J. Psycho-Anal.*, 70: 375–394.

Editor's Introduction to Chapter 9

Lawrence J. Brown

David Benhaim's chapter dealing with the origin and nature of Tradition is a perfect paper for the closing segment in this volume. He picks up Freud's (1939) query in *Moses*, "What the real nature of tradition resides in, and what its special power rests on" (p. 52). Additionally, how are we to understand the emergence of a tradition and its flourishing over centuries, even millennia? And, from a different perspective, how do some traditions disappear and lay fallow for centuries only to reappear after a long slumber – what Freud (1905) called the "return of the repressed"? Benhaim guides us through Freud's speculations of Akhenaten's monotheistic religion as the source of Moses' belief in one god; how the Pharoah's monotheism was overturned by the revanchist priesthood; then driven into obscurity (repressed) for many years until it reappeared (return of the repressed) in a new hybrid form. Benhaim discusses the subject of a *latency period* – first employed by Freud in his discussion of sexual development – as a factor in the development of an historical tradition. The 'latency period' familiar to psychoanalysts refers to a sexual repression in the *individual;* however, with respect to the development of a tradition, Benhaim describes a

> process of *collective latency* that is parallel with Freud's account of the murder of Moses… that of the Shoah (Holocaust) and the silence that followed before the event became an object of public debate.
>
> (this volume) (italics added)

Benhaim deepens the discussion of what constitutes a tradition by referencing Freud's distinction between the *oral tradition* and the *written tradition*, "What had been written or changed in the written record might very well have been preserved intact in oral tradition" (Freud, 1939, p. 68). Oral traditions, Freud comments, such as epic dramas handed down across the centuries, may be rooted in even a more long-forgotten event "which lies so far back, in such remote times, that only an obscure and incomplete tradition informs later generations of it (ibid., p. 71). Freud then bemoans that

DOI: 10.4324/9781003272045-18

> Surprise has been felt that the epic as an art-form has become extinct in later times… [and that] The old material has been used up and for all later events historical writing took the place of tradition.
>
> (p. 71)

Perhaps this lament captured Freud's dark mood ("The old material has been used up") as the grandeur of his beloved Vienna was invaded by the Nazis and the rich Jewish traditions were being destroyed? And we may wonder what long-forgotten events from our ancient histories are returning from repression today, being "remembered" through our current heroes? Are the gods from our ancient traditions waking from their repressed slumber to fuel today's superheroes with a clarity of what is right and wrong that seems to have been forgotten? Hopefully the old material has not been used up.

References

Freud, S. (1905) Three essays on the theory of sexuality. SE 7: 123–246.
Freud, S. (1939) Moses and Monotheism: Three Essays. SE 23: 1–138.

9 Freud

On Tradition

David Benhaim

How has the story of Moses's murder and of the original father survived over the ages? Also, how has the story of "his oblivion and of the decisive psychic and 'cultural' consequences of this murder" (Moscovici, 1991, p. 396) survived? These are the questions that plagued Freud in his last book *Moses and Monotheism*. To answer these questions, Freud introduced the link between latency and tradition: just as a child's Oedipal desires are repressed and then later return, so the murder of Moses, similarly repressed, comes back in new generations.

At the end of the second essay, Freud questions: "What the real nature of a tradition resides in, and what its special power rests on" (1939, p. 52). Yerushalmi, Derrida, Bernstein, and Assmann are the only ones who have seen this question as a key to understanding the third essay. Yerushalmi expresses it most clearly when he writes:

> Probably too absorbed by its sensational aspects – the Egyptianity of Moses and his murder by the Jews – readers of the Moses have generally failed to see that this book and, especially the third part, that crowns it, connects with the problem raised by the origin of tradition and most of all its dynamic.
>
> (1993, p. 73)

But, what does Freud mean by tradition? What is its origin, its dynamic, and ultimately the source of its power?

Freud's Notion of Tradition and the Return of the Repressed

Freud's understanding of tradition is implicit in his writings and this contribution examines his perspectives on the nature of tradition as gleaned from his works. Starting from his conclusion of the summary of the second essay, he highlights three important facts: **first** is the religion of Aten, a sun god, promulgated by the heretic Pharoah Akhenaten, who overthrew the existing Egyptian panoply of many gods and established the first

DOI: 10.4324/9781003272045-19

monotheistic religion in history. Akhenaten enforced Atenism as the state religion which created considerable turmoil in Egypt. At his death, Akhenaten's religion was abolished, and this period of Egyptian history sank into oblivion.

The **second** feature regarding Freud's concept of tradition derives from a man named Moses who was close to Akhenaten and an adherent of the pharaoh and his religion. This man, a follower of the religion of Aten, saw all his hopes vanish with Akhenaten's death and the abolition of Atenism. Finding himself unable to continue living in Egypt, he turned to foreigners of Semitic origin, left Egypt, and tried to realize his ideals with this new group. However, the precepts and laws that were imposed on them were too demanding. Thus, they rebelled against and murdered him, rejecting his religion. (Freud relied on the work of E. Sellin (1922), a historian, to support his premise of murder.)

The **third** fact relates to tribes that came out of Egypt and united with others with whom they had strong links. They settled in Meribat-Qades, an area rich in water. There, under the influence of the Arabian Midianites, they adopted a new religion whose volcanic god was called Yahweh and his priest Moses (a second individual named Moses). This god has no resemblance to the Mosaic god. The new religion was based on a compromise that recognized the claims of both sides: on one hand, those who wanted to deny the new and strange character of the god Yahweh and the increased submission he demanded of his people; on the other, those who wanted to maintain the memories of Egypt's liberation from slavery, of Moses's grandiose figure and of circumcision. To this was added "certain restrictions on the use of the name of the new god" (Freud, 1939, p. 62). Ed Meyer (1905) provides Freud support for this third fact. Subsequently, the episode of Moses, his murder and the monotheism seem to disappear. Freud tells us that "the remarkable thing, however, is that that was not the case – that the most powerful effects of the people's experience were to come to light only later and to force their way into reality in the course of many centuries" (1939, p. 62).

He emphasized that the transformation of Yahweh was a central fact in the later development of the Jewish religion, which lost its original characteristics and acquired those that resembled Aten, the ancient god of Moses. Thus, Akhenaten's monotheism reemerged after it's destruction, embodied as the ethical demand of a single God promulgated through the voice of the prophets. Freud ends this historical summary with a question that has two parts:

> Is there any need to call in the influence of Moses as a cause of the final form taken by the Jewish idea of God? It would not be enough to assume a spontaneous development to higher intellectuality during cultural life extending over hundreds of years?
>
> (1939, p. 64)

His answer revolves around two comments: in his first comment he suggests that the above explanation is not adequate. Indeed, in similar circumstances, the Greek people were not led toward monotheism, but toward the dissolution of polytheism and the beginnings of a constitution philosophical thought. In Egypt, monotheism was a collateral effect of imperialism; "God was a reflection of the Pharaoh who was the absolute ruler of a great world-empire" (Freud, 1939, p. 65). The political circumstances among the Jews were extremely unfavorable for allowing the transition from a national to a universal god. The idea of a chosen people would have remained quite problematic in this perspective. He concluded that "the problem of the origin of monotheism among the Jews would thus remain unsolved" (Freud, 1939, p. 65).

His second comment states that the Jewish chroniclers and historians show us, in a determined and uncontradictory way that the idea of a single god was brought to the Jews by Moses. This shows the will of the clergy to establish a continuity between Moses' religion and the subsequent Jewish religion, thus seeking to deny the *hiatus* that Freud has brought to light. The proposals put forward were therefore rejected, which led him to question the possible link between the latency period and tradition.

Latency Period and Tradition

Freud starts from an observation: three Mosaic doctrines had no echo among the common people: "the idea of a single god, the rejection of a magically effective ceremonial and the ethical demands" formulated in the name of that god. Only after a long interregnum did they begin to reappear and exert their presence. Freud then asked himself: "how are we to explain a delayed effect of this kind and where do we meet with a similar phenomenon?" (1939, p. 66). Three examples enabled him to elaborate his answer: **first**, Darwin's theory of evolution; **second,** the situation of an individual who acquires a new knowledge which he must recognize due to certain proofs that conflict with some of his most cherished desires and convictions; and, finally, a **third** – which Freud characterized as irrelevant – the case of a man who emerged unharmed from an accident –a railway collision – and who, in the following weeks developed a traumatic neurosis. Each of these examples has a *function*: the first two elaborate the notion of *affective resistances* and the necessity of sufficient time passing that enables the repressed to overcome the powerful forces of repression. The first, Darwin's theory, deals with the phenomenon of mass psychology; the second is its equivalent on the level of individual psychology. The third factor introduces us to the notion of *latency*. The articulation of these notions allows us to provide an explanation of the phenomenon. Freud asked what might be shared between traumatic neurosis and Jewish monotheism? *Latency*. According to the Freudian hypothesis, following Moses's murder and the abandonment of his religion, a long period elapsed during which no expression of the (Moses') monotheistic idea appears.

But what do we mean by latency? According to Laplanche and Pontalis, latency is the

> Period which extends from the dissolution of infantile sexuality (at the age of five or six) to the onset of puberty, constituting a pause in the evolution of sexuality. This stage sees a decrease in sexual activity, the desexualisation of object-relationships and of the emergence of such feelings as shame and disgust along with moral and aesthetic aspirations.
>
> According to psycho-analytic theory the latency period has its origin in the dissolution of the Oedipus complex; it represents an intensification of repression which brings about an amnesia affecting the earliest years, a transformation of object-cathexes into identifications with the parents, and a development of sublimations.
>
> (1973, p. 234)

This latency period results from the conflict between demands of the drives on the one hand and, on the other hand, the cultural demands. These put a brake on the drive demands which must adapt to them. Insofar as the latency period has its origin in the dissolution of the Oedipus complex, the infantile desire is confronted with the Oedipal prohibitions which set a limit. It is "in the space of a few years [that] the little primitive creature must turn into a civilized human being" (Freud, 1938, p. 185). The child becomes civilized by the constitution of barriers such as shame, disgust, but also by the emergence of moral and aesthetic aspirations and the development of sublimations. Freud transposes this period of latency at the collective level to the history of the people of Israel, amounting to the repression of the murder of Moses by an entire society: the individuals who comprise that group in addition to the entire society as well. According to Freud, this would cover the total period from the murder of Moses to the coming of the prophets who again manifest the features of Mosaic monotheism, particularly the conviction of a single God and the ethical demands formulated in the name of this God.

An example that could illustrate this process of collective latency that is parallel with Freud's account of the murder of Moses is that of the Shoah (Holocaust) and the silence that followed before the event became an object of public debate. As Eva Weil (2020) writes in her report:

> From the end of the Second World War and the catastrophe of Nazism, at least thirty years passed until the intertwining of their traces appeared in public debate. Further on, she adds: Taking the model of infantile latency as a starting point, latency in the collective would correspond to an apparently silent or almost silent time of thirty, forty,

> fifty years where few echoes of the catastrophe are heard, a time that is apparently empty and not very loud. The meaning, the movements and the character would appear only at the exit of this relative silence, by and in the very aftermath of its rupture. This analogy would offer an illumination for the time elapsed between the catastrophe of the Shoah and the appearance of multiple accounts, testimonies, and productions of all kinds a few decades later. This "latency" strongly influences individual and collective movements.[1]

Freud then returns to the Meribat-Qades compromise – the adoption of a new religion – to further explore the question of tradition:

> Both portions had the same interest in disavowing the fact of their having had an earlier religion and the nature of its content.
>
> (1939, p. 68)

The compromise was documented. Those who came from Egypt brought the knowledge of writing and the taste for historiography, but historiography did not yet recognize its obligation to tell the truth. As a result, "it had no scruples about shaping its narratives according to the needs and purposes of the moment, as though it had not yet recognized the concept of falsification" (Freud, 1939, p. 68). This is where the opposition comes into play between the *written fixation* and what Freud calls *tradition*, that is, "the oral transmission of the same material"[2] (1939, p. 68). It is essential to highlight Freud's primary concern with the *oral tradition* that he opposes to the *written fixation*.

Questioning their relationship, he develops the following paradox:

> What had been omitted or changed in the written record might very well have been preserved intact in tradition.
>
> (Freud, 1939, p. 68)

For Freud, the oral tradition appears simultaneously as the complement and the opposite of the written history. It seems to him to escape distortion, in part, and perhaps it escapes the distortion completely on certain points. In this sense, it would be more truthful than the written account. However, Freud does not hide his uncertainties about oral transmission given that it is less constant and precise than the written word. It is particularly subject to modifications and deformations, during intergenerational transmission. Such a tradition could know many outcomes: to be crushed by the written narration, to become more and more obscure and to finally become oblivious; but also, to end up in a written fixation "and especially, it can happen that it does not disappear as inscribed in the oral" (Moscovici, 2002, p. 135). This analysis rests on the analogy of what happens to the psychic life of an individual: the psychic events of early childhood know a similar course. During the latency period they will initially go in a subterranean and silent way only to reappear with force, sometimes with fracas, in adolescence or later in a distorted and displaced form, "but also in a more secret way, in phenomena of words and states of language, writes Marie Moscovici. In the sense of psychic reality, the truth would be inscribed in oral documents and not only in written unconscious archives" (Moscovici, 2002, p. 136).

How do these considerations apply to the latency of religious history? All that the official historiography has rejected has not been lost. This content has come to enrich the traditions of the people and to be preserved. Thus, according to Sellin – or, as Moscovici says,

> should we say, sheltered by Sellin's knowledge, who was a historian and could therefore seem to clear the excesses of imagination or wishful thinking to which Freud was happily prone.
>
> (Moscovici, 2002, p. 137)

A tradition about the murder of Moses would have survived, in priestly circles, which radically contradicted the official version and was closer to the truth. But, Freud objects, if it was known only to a few, "is that enough to explain its effect?" (Freud, 1939, p. 94). Does this knowledge, limited to the priestly caste of the Levites, have the power to captivate the masses as soon as they become aware of it? His hypothesis is that among the ignorant masses there must be something that resembles this lost knowledge and is in some way similar to the learning of the few. Marie Moscovici considers this the introduction of a new distinction: she notes the difference between written fixation and oral transmission and views them from a sociological perspective. The written word is the prerogative of the Levites who constituted the priestly caste. It is matched by the orality of the "people" which does not constitute knowledge.

> And it is from their encounter, when they come together, that the strength of recollection, or the return of the repressed, is born, attesting to the obvious presence of elements, of traces, of the most remote past.
>
> (Moscovici, 2002, p. 138)

Freud insisted on the strength of these traditions:

> The remarkable fact is that these traditions, instead of becoming weaker with time, became more and more powerful in the course of centuries, forced their way into the later revisions of the official accounts and finally showed themselves strong enough to have a decisive influence on the thoughts and actions of people.
>
> (Freud, 1939, p. 69)

Freud speaks both of *tradition* in the singular and *traditions* in the plural. A distinction that Ricœur elaborated in *Time and Narrative* that allows us to clarify Freud's views. Tradition would be "the instance of legitimacy" and would designate "the claim to the truth whereas traditions consist in the transmitted contents as carriers of meaning; they place all the received heritages in the order of the symbolic and, virtually, in a linguistic and textual dimension; as such, **the traditions are proposals of meaning**" (Ricœur, 1985, p. 410). He insists on the notion of an *heir* that is ours and on the determining role the linguistic dimension plays in the transmission: The notion of tradition, taken in the sense of traditions, means that we are never in an absolute position as innovators, but at first are indebted to the teachings of our heirs. This condition is essentially due to the linguistic structure of communication in general and of the transmission of past contents in particular. Language is the great institution – the institution of institutions – that has always preceded us. And by language we mean not only the language system in every natural language, but "the things already said, heard and received. By tradition we mean therefore the things already said," as they are transmitted to us along the chains of interpretation and reinterpretation (Ricœur, 1985, p. 400). This way of conceiving tradition also allows us to introduce the notion of *the work of tradition* which we see in the text of Freud quoted above. It would be something comparable to *dream work* or to the work of *mourning* which is characterized by a process of transformation and reappropriation that allows these traditions, as Freud said, to "force their way into the later revisions of the official accounts." (Freud, 1939, p. 69).

What circumstances produced this result?

Freud traces the evolution of Jewish religious history: he recalls the abandonment of the religion of Aten after the murder of Moses – that he does not address – in favor of the cult of Yahweh: the skewed tendencies that he discovered at work in the Bible constituted an attempt by the official narrative to hide this shameful fact. Finally, we witness the return of the abandoned Mosaic religion. However, we see that the religion of Moses has left traces:

> Some sort of memory of it was kept alive – a possibly obscured and distorted tradition. And it was this tradition of a great past that continued to operate (from the background, as it were), that gradually acquired more and more power over people's minds and which in the end succeeded in changing the god Yahweh into the Mosaic god and in re-awakening into life the religion of Moses that had been introduced and then abandoned long centuries before.
>
> (Freud, 1939, 70)

"What about this 'kind of memory'"? asks Marie Moscovici. It is deposited in the oral, even if, according to Freud, it will then be anchored in the writing of tales, legends, and epics. She qualifies *these memories as* marranos memories. The narrative forms these memories will continue to be transmitted, like underground currents, deformed, obscured, but we will be able to find them,

> or at least to find some clues, some vestiges. They will be conducting threads for the eyes that read and perhaps especially for the ears that listen. It is not neutral [...] that the main themes around which all these memory relics mobilized Freud were, for him, the idea of the repressed murder of Moses, a hidden repetition of the murder of the father, and that of circumcision, the "guiding fossil" of a castration once accomplished.[3]
>
> (Moscovici, 2002, p. 137)

This religion of Moses would have been preserved in the form of an oral tradition, *obscured and deformed*, and would have continued to act in the transformation of the god Yahweh into the image of the god of Moses who would thus have made a strong comeback. It is indeed the model of repression, latency, and the return of the repressed. Freud concluded by saying:

> That a tradition thus sunk in oblivion should exercise such a powerful effect on the mental life of a people is an unfamiliar idea to us.
>
> (1939, p. 70)

Freud wonders, "where do we feel at home?" He links this query to his studies of mass psychology in order to explain the problem (Porte, 1999, p. 220). Michèle Porte rightly points out that mass psychology is a field that Freud has been working on for a quarter of a century: how can he then speak of unfamiliarity? She asks:

> Isn't there a displacement? Is it not this analysis of the history of a mass – Jewish history of religion – that creates in Freud the feeling, then more understandable, of the uncanny of not being from the country?
>
> (Porte, 1999, p. 81)

In response to her question, Porte notes that Freud turned to his earlier studies on mass psychology, as shown in his interest of Greek history and culture, which he literally visited in order to explore other sceneries. The analogy with the Greek people allowed Freud to conclude that epics such as the *Iliad* and the *Odyssey* are traces of epochs "of external brilliance and cultural efflorescence" (1939, p. 70) that have been preserved in *an obscure tradition* and are called to life through poetry. In *Group Psychology and the Analysis of the Ego*, Freud recognized the poet's capacity to create the first ego ideal and to detach itself from the masses (Scarfone, 1999, pp. 188–189).

For Freud, epic poetry is linked to tradition that initially is constituted as an oral transmission prior to being anchored in writing:

> National epics of other peoples – Germans, Indians, Finns – have come to light as well. It is the business of historians of literature to investigate whether we may assume the same determinants for their origin as with the Greeks. Such an investigation would, I believe, yield a positive result. Here is the determinant which we recognize: a piece of prehistory which, immediately after it, would have been bound to appear rich in content, important, splendid, and always, perhaps, heroic, but which lies so far back, in such remote times, that only an obscure and incomplete tradition informs later generations of it. Surprise has been felt that the epic as an art-form has become extinct in later times. The explanation may be that its determining cause no longer exists. The old material was used up and for all later events historical writing took the place of tradition. The greatest heroic deeds of our days have not been able to inspire an epic, and even Alexander the Great had a right to complain that he would found no Homer.
>
> (1939, p. 71)

In this context, the epic poet is the one who reinvigorates through his poems the obscure historical memories carried by tradition. "One might almost say, writes Freud, that the vaguer tradition has become, the more serviceable it becomes for a poet" (1939, p. 71). however, the epic poetry disappears when historiography takes the place of the tradition. In this connection, Moscovici wonders about

> the fate of the figure of the hero or the poet when the heroism of the life of heroes cannot be linked to the previous generations, to the collective "fathers" – or even to some personal fathers? Can the "primal scenes" of contemporary generations, its wars whose frightening victories often left a taste of defeat, be in the imaginary as they were in the previous century? One sometimes even has the feeling that today, in psychoanalysis, a lot of work is needed so that the "primal scene" itself, this pillar of our theories and our practice, finds again or finds, if one dares to say, the taste that it had. All nostalgia aside if that is possible.
>
> (2002, p. 217)

According to Freud, this reflection on epic poetry and tradition makes us more apt to accept this "strange hypothesis: that it was the tradition of Moses which, for the Jews, altered the worship of Yahweh in the direction of the old Mosaic religion" (1939, p. 72).

We have here the same tradition which in one situation is transformed into an epic and in the other into a religion. How can we understand that the same tradition gives rise to two such different results, unless we see religion as an immense poem and the Jewish religion – as the epic of the history of the Jewish people? Freud admits the impotence of the oral tradition to explain the survival of the story of the murder of Moses – and, beyond that, of the murder of the original father – of its oblivion and of the decisive psychic and cultural consequences of this murder. He concludes his analysis by affirming that

> a tradition that was based only on communication could not lead to the compulsive character that attaches to religious phenomena. It would be listened to, judged, and perhaps dismissed, like any other piece of information from the outside; it would never attain the privilege of being liberated from the constraint of logical thought.[4]
>
> (Freud, 1939, p. 101)

Is this an admission of failure? Under what conditions would tradition be likely to shed light on religious phenomena and the constraints that characterizes them? What path should such a tradition follow?

The Archaic Heritage

To answer these questions, Freud started from the observation that the psychic life of the individual juxtaposes contents experienced by oneself along with others transmitted at birth, elements of phylogenetic origin, what he calls an *archaic heritage*. He thus introduces the *phylogenetic hypothesis* which runs across his work. Starting with Chapter VII of *The Interpretation of Dreams* to the *Outline of Psychoanalysis, Totem and Taboo, The Claims of Psychoanalysis to Scientific Interest, The Wolf Man, The Ego and the Id, Moses and Monotheism*, Freud does not stop reinitiating, rethinking, and rearticulating themes of memory and transmission, always insisting on their provisional character. Freud never developed these themes in a complete explanatory or demonstrative mode. According to the word of Marie Moscovici, *The Epic of the Mind* – it's the way she calls the phylogenetic hypothesis – constituted for him a conviction from which he would never withdraw. It is one of the cornerstones of the psychoanalytical edifice. In his work, *The Claims of Psychoanalysis to Scientific Interest*, he states:

> In the last few years, psychoanalytic writers have become aware that the principle that "ontogeny is a repetition of phylogeny" must be applicable to mental life, and this has led to a fresh extension of psychoanalytic interest.
>
> (1913b, p. 184)

This fundamental biogenetic principle, obvious to Freud and his contemporaries, was formulated by the zoologist Haeckel, who spread Darwin's theories in Germany. For Haeckel, ontogeny is the individual development of the living being and phylogeny the counterpart for the species. For Freud, psychoanalysis constituted an attempt to transpose this principle to the level of psychic life and to try to understand and reconstruct, next to the individual psychic development, that of the species as it is expressed through the individual psyche. What use does Freud make of this principle? How does he insert it into psychoanalysis? He has recourse to it at precise moments of psychoanalytic explanation. In the story of *The Wolf Man*, he takes care to underline its methodological and clinical use. In contrast to Jung, Freud emphasizes the clinical importance and the primacy of the explanation of ontogeny; he insists on the necessity of first exhausting all the possibilities of ontogeny before resorting to the phylogenetic explanation. This model inspired Freud to assert that the *archaic heritage* is primarily that of the instinct. Instincts are, for him, the repositories of the experiences of the species, as if animals kept memories of what their ancestors had experienced. This explains why, in his eyes, faced with new life situation, the animal can behave as if it were an old and familiar situation. In man, the archaic heritage would correspond to the instincts of the animals, but with a much more diversified scope and content. However, as Marie Moscovici rightly points out, we are dealing with a metaphor of instincts, an analogy that allows Freud to make his idea understood and advanced, rather than with a theory of an anatomical-physiological setup. But this first approach, which allows us to situate the archaic heritage in relation to the instincts, remains insufficient if it is not completed by an analysis of its content. What else does this heritage consist of? Freud clearly distinguished two elements: *dispositions* and *contents*, that is to say, mnemonic traces of what previous generations have experienced (Freud, 1939, p. 99). What are these dispositions?

In the preface to the third edition of the *Three Essays on the Theory of Sexuality*, Freud distinguished the accidental from the dispositional. The accidental refers to the events experienced in early childhood, whereas the dispositional constitutes a kind of sedimentation that takes shape from the previous experiences of the species. The sum of these two factors creates the disposition as an ability to react in a particular way to excitations and impressions and, for development, to evolve in certain directions.

The second element, memory traces, outlines a theory of collective memory from the notions of universality of language symbolism and tradition as well as reactions to early traumas. The universal symbolism of language is present in dreams and is common in children who symbolically represent a thing or an act by another, without having been taught to do so. Despite the diversity of languages, this universal symbolism is the same for all peoples. Freud speculated that we are dealing here with an original but forgotten language (Freud, 1939, p. 99). With respect to the impact of early traumas, while their effects are experienced in accord with the individual's psychic organization, symptomatic reactions may seem to move away from the original experience and are organized by a phylogenetic model. Freud takes the example of the Oedipal and Castration complexes in which the individual reactions seem unjustified if they are not considered in relation to the lived experience of previous generations. He compares this to putting one's clothes into already used baggage (Freud, 1939, p. 99).

Tradition and Memory

For Freud, the notion of tradition is interwoven with his thoughts about memory. Freud disagrees with the rejection by biological science of his thesis that acquired characteristics may be genetically transmitted across generations. However, as he points out, it is indispensable for psychoanalytical work. What does Freud mean by tradition? In his view, it is formed from the acquired inheritances which are constructed from transmitted contents as carriers of meaning. Furthermore, tradition is characterized by direct oral communication and by the transmission of conscious memories conveyed from grandparents to grandchildren through storytelling of shared experiences. Freud also asserts that the heredity and transmission of mnemonic traces from experiences of previous generations are also transmitted, independent of any direct communication or educational influence between these separate generations. But, in contrast to the claims of the biological scientists, could we argue that we are dealing with an essentially biological memory since it depends entirely on the transmission of acquired characteristics to the descendants? Freud seems to have anticipated this objection when he clearly underlined the difference between biological and psychic.

However, the centrality of the psyche remains for Freud his primary preoccupation, especially when he approaches the questions of transmission and conservation of archaic experiences or even when he borrows from biology. In this regard, Freud wrote:

> The same thing is not in question, indeed, in the two cases: in the one it is a matter of acquired characters which are hard to grasp, in the other of memory-traces of external events – something tangible, as it were. But it may well be that at bottom we cannot imagine one without the other.
>
> (1939, p. 100)

It is a question of two types of memory or, to use an expression of Derrida, of *transgenerational archive* (1995); the mnemonic trace of an ancestral experience or the biologically acquired character, something like a memory of the organism. The hypothesis of the conservation of the mnemonic traces makes it possible to create a bridge between individual psychology and collective psychology, that of the masses, and to treat the people like individuals. Derrida comments on this passage:

> All that Freud says is that we are receptive to an analogy between the two types of transgenerational memory or archive (the memory of an ancestral experience or the so-called biologically acquired character) and that "we cannot imagine [vorstellen] one without the other" [SE 23: 100]. Without the irrepressible, that is to say, only suppressible and repressible, force and authority of this transgenerational memory, the problems of which we speak would be dissolved and resolved in advance. There would no longer be any essential history of culture, there would no longer be any question of memory and of archive, of patriarchive or of matriarchive, and one would no longer even understand how an ancestor can speak within us, nor what sense there might be in us to speak to him or her, to speak in such an "unheimlich," "uncanny" fashion, to his or her ghost. With it.
>
> (1995, p. 59)

The Archaic Heritage and Its Evidence

What evidence does Freud offer to support these notions of an archaic inheritance? As he himself states, the only evidence he can put forward is that of "the residual phenomena of the work of analysis which calls for a phylogenetic derivation," (1939, p. 100) which seems to Freud an obvious and solid perspective. What are these *"residual phenomena"* of analytic work? Marie Moscovici refers to these residues as past events. We can say these residues constitute the daily material of analytic work: dreams, parapraxes, symptoms, but also, myths, tales, and especially the language itself insofar as this material only takes shape in it and through it. It is these residues that are the carriers of long forgotten events that are transmitted from one generation to the next. The history that they reveal is not one transmitted through writing; rather, it is one that is inscribed, deposited without the knowledge of its bearer and which remains, so to speak, separate from official history (Moscovici, 1991, p. 394). It is through this perspective that we may understand this curious affirmation of Freud:

> I have no hesitation in declaring that men have always known (in this special way) that they once possessed a primal father and killed him.
>
> (1939, p. 101)

Children at play innately "know" about primal fathers and their murder by the child himself and this knowledge, simultaneously known but not known, easily vanishes when the toys are put away. Forgetting is the way to protect the memory, to preserve it. But what forgetting are we talking about? Repression removes the sense of ownership and creates a memory that is not the one we designate by "I"; instead, it is a memory that we no longer consciously own. Repression preserves the event and inscribes it in an indelible impersonal way, so that we can no longer speak about memories in the usual sense of conscious awareness. Freud's original technique in *The Studies on Hysteria* focused on the goal of unearthing the buried/repressed memory, revealed through hypnosis as a reminiscence, thereby making the unconscious conscious and allowing the memory to be revealed as an aspect of "I."

Memory-Traces: Conservation and Transmission

Since we are dealing with archaic heritage, we are entitled to ask ourselves where the mnemonic traces are preserved and how they are transmitted. In the last pages of *Totem and Taboo*, Freud formulated two assumptions that were implicit in his previous analyses. The first, foundational for his thinking about the memory traces of archaic heritage, is that of a collective mind, similar to the psychic life of an individual, in which psychic processes are accomplished. This hypothesis is indispensable to him to explain the perpetuation of feelings of guilt over the centuries and generations that were unaware of the primal father's murder. Without this continuity there would be neither progress nor evolution, each new generation would have to start again, to acquire all that the previous generations have acquired. Freud then raised two questions. The first one concerns the part attributed to the psychic continuity in the sequence of generations; the second one concerned the ways and means used by a generation to transmit its psychic states to the next one. His answer specified two things: tradition as ordinarily understood, that is, as direct transmission, is discarded because it does not bring a satisfactory answer, as we have shown. It is rather the heredity of the psychic dispositions which ensures this continuity; however, to be enabled, they need to be stimulated by individual life. The words of Goethe's Faust seem relevant here:

> What thou hast inherited from thy fathers, acquire it to make it thine.
> (Goethe, 1984, p. 45)

Freud wants to underline that the reception of the inheritance is not passive, and it requires the active engagement of the subject to appropriate it. René Kaës sees in this aphorism the division of the inheriting subject as the subject of the unconscious. This subject is divided between a double necessity; he writes

> a twofold existence: one to serve his own purposes and the other as a link in a chain, which he serves against his will, or at least involuntarily.
> (Freud, 1914, p. 78)

Freud formulates this double division in a very clear way in *Totem and Taboo* when he considers the question of narcissism. He keenly observes that the narcissism of the infant is supported by that of the previous generation: the generation of the parents who transmit to the infant the dreams that they were unable to accomplish along with the wish and the firm conviction that he will accomplish them. Freud then introduces – this will be his second assumption – a curious hypothesis which will not appear again in any of his works; indeed, he will never take it up again nor discuss it:

> For psychoanalysis has shown that everyone possesses in his unconscious mental activity an apparatus which enables him to interpret other people's reactions, that is, to undo the distortions which other people have imposed on the expression of their feelings.
>
> (Freud, 1913a, p. 159)

It is, as René Kaës affirms, the unconscious apparatus of transmission. By the unconscious comprehension that it allows, it plays a crucial role in the transmission of the affective inheritance to the later generations, inheritance resulting from "all the customs, ceremonies, and prescriptions that the primitive relationship to the primal father had left behind." (Kaës, 1989, p. 197). This second hypothesis raises questions that, as René Kaës points out, await answers that Freud perhaps never considered; mainly those that concern the constitution and functioning of this apparatus as well as its modality of transmission, namely the possible modification of what is transmitted. Kaës, for his part, alludes to Bion and his work on the apparatus for thinking thoughts as well as to the alpha function as concepts that allow us to clarify Freud's hypothesis.

Conclusion

As psychoanalysts, we cannot get rid of this prodigious speculative construction by considering it as absurd because its biological foundation is erroneous. We are obliged, as we would do with one of our patients, to ask ourselves what its function in Freud's approach is and how we may rethink it today as a potentially heuristic tool to assist us in our practice as well as in our theoretical elaborations. We can conceive it as a fiction or a metaphor that helps us to think about the links between the subject and his ancestors; to consider what survives in us and weighs on our lives; what they did not manage to elaborate, but which they transmitted to us. This is what we often struggle with, living with something strange and foreign that haunts us, but that we do not manage to understand and even less to elaborate. The essential question that led Freud to construct the phylogenetic fantasy is an exemplary illustration: it is the question of guilt that organizes culture: a guilt linked to an original fault. How do we explain the persistence of this guilt through the centuries and millennia?

The constructions elaborated in *Totem and Taboo* – primitive horde, association of the sons, murder of the father, ambivalence of the feelings, totemic meal – create a model on which the beginning of civilization is based. It should be noted that the phylogenetic fantasy is first associated in Freud's work with the reflection on *Kultur*, a dimension of his work that contemporary psychoanalysts have abandoned, considering it wrongly as marginal and without clinical relevance, whereas he never ceases to repeat that *Kultur* and neurosis are indissociable.

The phylogenetic fantasy has the function of showing the vicissitudes of guilt and how it is transmitted. In the end, we can conceive it as a fantasy of psychic transmission. What this transmission reveals to us is the passage from material reality, the reality of fact, to psychic reality. The events that were initially played out on an external stage have ended up being played out on the internal stage. In other words, the psychic reality has a foundation in the collective history to which we all have belonged long before our birth: as Piera Aulagnier would say, conceived by our parents but itself infiltrated, without their knowledge, by the history of our ancestors. Faced with certain patients, we sometimes have the impression that, like Oedipus, their life obeys an oracle whose meaning we can only understand insofar as we find identificatory traits belonging to previous generations. The analysis of the phylogenetic fantasy teaches us, on the one hand, that transmission is ensured by inherited psychic dispositions but stimulated by individual life events; on the other hand, that the interpretation apparatus allows us to appropriate what comes to us from previous generations and to transform it. Finally, as in the case of the murder of the primal father, transmission is based on the repetition of events.

Notes

1 For the notion of collective latency and its elaboration, I refer to the remarkable report by Eva Weil in Weil Eva, Lieux du traumatique, le génocide: le nouage collectif-individuel, Bulletin de la SPP, 2020.

2 I would like to make two points:

1. This distinction that Freud makes between the written and the oral cannot fail to recall what in Jewish tradition is known as the Written Torah and the Oral Torah, both given to Moses on Sinai, the latter being the explanation of the former. It is the Oral Torah that will be the source of the Talmud and which will end up, after the second Exile, being written down. Does Freud take up this distinction when he speaks of written fixation and oral transmission of the same event? In any case, Jewish tradition already offers him the distinction.
2. In her book *Le meurtre et la langue*, Métailié, 2002, Marie Moscovici writes about the double face of this very word: oral. The oral, that which passes through the mouth, food, or speech, that enters or leaves it (as well as

speech that enters, food which leaves), involvement of the eating and the speaking, which makes the mouth a vital and symbolic dimension, of need and desire, of absorption and expression, place of essential production (p. 154).

3 The Marrano metaphor of memory could not be more relevant, if we consider that the example of the Marranos of Spain and Portugal constitutes a flawless illustration of the tradition as Freud sees it.

4 Ibid., p. 101.

References

Derrida, J. (1995), *Mal d'Archive*, Paris, Galilée.

Freud, S. (1905), *Three Essays on the Theory of Sexuality*. Standard Edition, 7: 125–243. London: Hogarth Press, 1964.

Freud, S. (1913a), *Totem and Taboo*. Standard Edition, 13: 1–161. London: Hogarth Press, 1964.

Freud, S. (1913b), *The Claims of Psychoanalysis to Scientific Interest*. Standard Edition, 13: 165–190. London: Hogarth Press, 1964

Freud, S. (1914), *On Narcissism: An introduction*. Standard Edition, 14: 69–102. London: Hogarth Press, 1964

Freud, S. (1921), *Group Psychology and Analysis of the Ego*. Standard Edition, 18: 67–143. London: Hogarth Press, 1964.

Freud, S. (1939), *Moses and Monotheism, Three Essays*. Standard Edition, 23:1–137. London: Hogarth Press, 1964.

Freud, S. (1940 [1938]), *An Outline of Psychoanalysis*. Standard Edition, 23: 141–207. London: Hogarth Press, 1964.

Goethe, J. W. von (1832), *Faust I et II*, Garnier-Flammarion, 1984.

Kaës, R. (1989), *Ruptures catastrophiques et travail de la mémoire*. In: *Violence d'État et psychanalyse*, ed. René Kaëset Janine Puget. Paris, Dunod, pp. 169–204.

Laplanche, J. & Pontalis, J. B. (1973), *The Language of Psychoanalysis*, 1–497, The International Psycho-analytic Library. Pep-Web.org

Meyer, E. (1905), *Die Mosessagen und die Lewiten*, S.B.Akad.Wiss.Berl. (Phil.-Hist. Kl.) 31,640.

Moscovici, M. (1991), *Il est arrivé quelque chose*, Paris, Payot.

Moscovici, M. (2002), *Le meurtre et la langue*, Paris, Métailié.

Porte, M. (1999), *Le Mythe monothéiste*, Paris, ENS Éditions.

Ricœur, P. (1985), *Temps et récit, III, Le temps raconté*. Paris, Seuil, Essais.

Scarfone, D. (1999), *Oublier Freud?* Montréal, Boréal.

Sellin, E. (1922), *Mose und seine Bedeutung für die israelitische-jüdische Religiongeschichte*, Leipzig.

Weil, E. (2020) *Lieux du traumatique, le génocide: le nouage collectif-individuel*. Revue Française de Psychanalyse 2021/5 (Vol.85), PUF.

Yerushalmi, Y. H. (1993), *Le Moïse de Freud, Judaïsme terminable et interminable*, Gallimard, NRF Essais.

Conclusion and Final Thoughts

Lawrence J. Brown

As Editor, I found myself unsure of what to address in this concluding chapter. Have there been issues raised that I could expand upon or, perhaps, some important topics that had not been given sufficient attention in these chapters? As I pondered this question, a song (1998) by the folk-rock singer Eric Andersen, *Rain Falls Down in Amsterdam*, suddenly meandered into my mind. I had not heard the song for several years and it appeared now as a *reverie* that captured and represented the emotions launched by the artist's song. The song by Andersen was a departure from his usual softer melodies: an angry one that depicts the sense of an unending repetitive European horror: the devastation of World War I, the failed Treaty of Versailles, and the incremental build-up to Naziism leading inexorably to World War II and the Holocaust. These associations to the song made me aware that the impact of the rise of Naziism on Freud and psychoanalysis required some elaboration. This has been an interest of mine, specifically with regard to the impact of the rise of Naziism on Freud and psychoanalysis.

In addition, I have a longstanding interest in the Pharoah Akhenaten (Amenhotep IV) who plays a central role in Freud's speculation that Moses had borrowed Akhenaten's monotheistic beliefs and built on these to create the monotheism of the Israelites. These two topics – the impact of Naziism in the 1930's on Freud and the influence of Akhenaten on Moses' monotheism – are discussed in the following pages. Both Freud and Akhenaten are readily identified with the cities in which they lived – Freud in Vienna and Akhenaten in the capital he built, Akhetaten/Amarna – and their connections to their respective cities are considered here. What follows is not intended to be an extensive review of these topics, but rather an overview of subjects that are essential to the background of *Moses and Monotheism*.

DOI: 10.4324/9781003272045-20

A Tale of Two Cities: Vienna and Akhetaten (Amarna)

Vienna: Coming of the Second World War

In 1931 the Permanent Committee for Literature and the Arts of the League of Nations invited Albert Einstein to dialogue in an exchange of letters with a person and subject of his choosing. Einstein, a lifelong pacifist, troubled by the frightening portent of Hitler's National Socialist Party, its antisemitic language and bellicosity, proposed a relevant topic for their correspondence: Einstein initiated the discussion in a letter to Freud (July 30, 1932) in which he asked, "Is there any way of delivering mankind from the menace of war?," and added that

> It is common knowledge that, with the advance of modern science, this issue has come to mean *a matter of life and death for civilization as we know it.*[1]
>
> (1933 [1932], p. 199) (italics added)

Regarding such brutality, Einstein wrote Freud that he pinned his hopes for the future on the kind of international organization such as the League of Nations that would be empowered to intercede in international conflicts; however, he realized that such organizations are composed of men and are limited

> Because man has within him a lust for hatred and destruction. In normal times this passion exists in a latent state, it emerges only in unusual circumstances; but it is a comparatively easy task to call it into play and raise it to the power of a collective psychosis. Here lies, perhaps, the crux of all the complex of factors we are considering, an enigma that only the expert [Freud] in the lore of human instincts can resolve.
>
> (op cit, p. 200)

Freud had already given this topic thought and had written a paper on the subject of war, "Thoughts for the Times on War and Death" (1915), composed in the midst of the First World War, and replied a month later to Einstein:

> Musing on the atrocities recorded on history's page, we feel that the ideal motive [i. e. "good war"] has often served as a camouflage for the lust of destruction; sometimes, as with the cruelties of the Inquisition, it seems that, while the ideal motives occupied the foreground of

> consciousness, they drew their strength from the destructive instincts submerged in the unconscious.
>
> (1933, SE 22, p. 210)

Laurence Kahn (this volume) recounts the bleakness of this period in her paper, "The Probable in Nazi Times," and begins her essay with a brief and potent comment, "*The Man Moses and the Monotheistic Religion* is a book of despair… infinitely deeper than that which followed the destruction of the second Temple in Jerusalem by Titus" in 70 AD.[2] Kahn does not mention the earlier first Temple, built by King Solomon, which was razed by the Babylonian King Nebuchadnezzar II, resulting in the exile of large numbers of Jews into far flung communities. Has Kahn overlooked this repetition? But perhaps her statement that there is an anguish "infinitely deeper" leaves the reader to ponder some other offense that is even more devastating than these actions: the rise of Hitler's Naziism and its attempts to rid the world of all traces of the Jewish people. In one of his more searing observations of humanity Freud observed that culture and society could easily be overturned and that we live in a time that was a "specially remarkable period… [in which] we find to our astonishment that *progress has allied itself with barbarism*" (Freud, 1939, p. 156) (italics added). This comment added to his despair about humanity when he wrote to Arnold Zweig (1927) that "I find myself confirmed in my wholly non-scientific belief that mankind on the average are a wretched lot" (p. 15).

As a possible Second World War loomed likely and Hitler's army gobbled up more swaths of territory for *lebensraum*,[3] Freud was confronted with a necessary decision that reiterated his ancestors' flight from anti-Semitic persecution in the Middle Ages (Freud, 1925). As the Nazi encroachment of his beloved Vienna made remaining there dangerous to his family, himself, and psychoanalysis, he understood the necessity of emigrating to the United Kingdom. 1937 was a very hard year for Freud in which he was recovering from two exceptionally painful surgeries of his jaw, and it became very clear that there was an active cancer. In addition, he learned of the death of Lou Andreas-Salome who was an important colleague and confidant of Freud's and this loss was compounded by his fear of a Nazi invasion of Austria which brought on a pique of despair:

> My only hope is that I shall not live to see it. It is a similar situation to 1681 when the Turks were besieging Vienna… If our town falls, the Prussian barbarians will flood over Europe.
>
> (Letter to Ernest Jones, 2/3/1937)

However, this wish was not to come true and Freud had to witness the Nazi Anschluss into his cherished Vienna on March 12, 1938, six months before his death on September 23, 1939.

However, Freud, now 81 years old and ill with cancer, persevered and wrote two important papers,[4] as well as continuing to complete his writing *Moses and Monotheism*, which Yerushalmi (1991, p. 2) perceptively stated that "the book can be read as a final chapter in Freud's lifelong case history."

Freud was no stranger to the savagery of mankind and fully understood the inherent cruelty that resides in all of us, but there was nothing more punishing for him than the day four armed Gestapo officers came to his door to arrest Anna and took her away for "questioning." For some unrealistic reason, the Nazis feared that the International Psychoanalytic Association had plotted to undermine the Third Reich and so interrogating her was necessary. In addition, "the Gestapo told her they had information about a conspiracy of Jewish ex-soldiers who were about to terrorize Vienna" (Cohen, 2012, p. 175). The bizarreness of these accusations notwithstanding, Freud, at home in the company of SS soldiers ransacking his apartment looking for hidden Jewish treasure, was terrified the Nazis might torture Anna. He paced the floor for what must have felt like an eternity, smoking his cigars, until she was returned several hours later. Unbeknownst to him, Anna had asked their family physician, Max Schur, for several pills of the poisonous Veronal for her brother, Martin, and herself in case they were to be tortured.

Freud's frightening confrontation with the Gestapo collided with his conception of a '*process of civilization*' (Freud, 1930) (italics added) which had two precepts: "strengthening of intellectual life" and the "renunciation of instinct," which clearly stood in opposition to the brutality and narrow mindedness of the Nazis. Freud extensively discussed the gradual evolution of a society in *Civilization and Its Discontents* (ibid.) and stated:

> that the inclination to aggression is an original, self-subsisting instinctual disposition in man… [and in] my view that it constitutes the greatest impediment to civilization
>
> (ibid., p. 122)

Matthia Beier (2020) expands on Freud's 'process of civilization' and ties the aggression of anti-Semitism to the concept of *Geistigkeit*, a German word that is difficult to translate into English, but is approximated by the notion of *intellectuality* that is in opposition to unbridled *sensuality*. In Beier's view, this distinction is related to anti-Semitism and he notes Freud's two thoughts about the source of anti-Semitism: (1) the oppression of sensuality and emphasis on intellectuality/spirituality and (2) reaction to the Jewish covenant with God and the notion that they are a chosen people in God's eyes. Furthermore, Beier states that anti-Semitism is magnified "as a 'blowback against monotheism,' [and in particular] against the Jewish peoples' form of *Geistigkeit* (intellectuality) and the notion of exclusive chosenness" (pp. 3–4).

Amarna: The Birth of Monotheism

[I ask the reader's forbearance if my remarks in this section seem slanted in a particular direction: I must confess that I am an Akhenaten-phile and have been since late adolescence after reading the book, *The Egyptian*, by Mika Waltari and also seeing the film on which it was based. I have read extensively and with much curiosity about the Pharoah and his family, and wrote my first psychoanalytic (unpublished) paper, "A Psychoanalytic Study of the Pharoah Akhenaten," while I was a post-doctoral fellow at the Menninger Clinic in the mid-1970s. Coincidentally, the head of the Topeka Psychoanalytic Institute was a Coptic Egyptian, Ishak Ramzey, and we had interesting discussions about Egypt, it's very long history and, of course, about psychoanalysis.]

In the Introduction to this book, I examined Freud's deep identification with Moses, beginning with his reverence for the prophet and preoccupying his childhood years. The question of who Moses was to Freud has also been considered in these papers, including a kind of twinship between them as leaders (of the Israelites and of the psychoanalytic movement).

Whether Moses was an actual historical or a fictional person is rarely raised in these essays, and Assmann's (2014) distinction between Moses and Akhenaten is helpful in this regard:

> Akhenaten is a figure of history without memory, Moses is a figure of memory without history.
>
> (Ibid., p. 61)

In 1934 Freud wrote to his close friends, Lou Andreas Salome and Arnold Zweig, and asked,

> One wonders how the Jew came to be what he is and why he attracted this undying hatred,

to which Freud concluded, "Moses created the Jewish *character*"[5] (italics added). In this comment, Freud appeared to view Moses as a sort of transformational figure:

> the Hebrews were only transformed into a veritable people or nation when God liberated them through Moses from their Egyptian bondage and formed a new covenant based on detailed legislation.
>
> (Ibid., p. 46)

Freud asserted that monotheism was not created by Moses, but rather that Moses 'borrowed' Akhenaten's type of monotheism and further elaborated it to create his own version (see below).

At first view, the limestone walls of the Valley of the Kings in Egypt appear to be dotted with numerous dark spots which upon closer inspection are the excavated entryways into the tombs and burial chambers of the Pharaohs, their families, and high-ranking nobles. These burial sites were well hidden in numerous locations throughout the Valley, but determined grave robbers unearthed most of these tombs and over the centuries plundered the priceless riches contained in the vaults. European expeditions began in earnest with French and English excursions at the close of the eighteenth century, journeys that revealed the bountiful treasures of ancient Egyptian culture; however, these same discoveries also triggered extensive looting and a massive transfer of antiquities to European museums and individuals. Additional excavations continued throughout the nineteenth century and the American explorer, Theodore Davis, announced in 1912 that "I fear that the Valley of Kings is now exhausted" – yet only a decade later Howard Carter discovered the intact burial site of the young king Tutankhamen in the Valley.

The unmolested display of priceless riches contained in Tutankhamen's tomb dazzled the world, but the *attention of psychoanalysts* was directed toward the young king's father, Akhenaten (formerly known as Amenhotep IV). Amenhotep III reigned over Egypt for roughly 39 years, a time of great prosperity, strength, and architectural achievements. He married a commoner who became his Great Royal Wife, Queen Tiye, and they had two sons and four daughters. One of his sons predeceased his father and the other rose to the throne at 12 years old as Amenhotep IV upon his father's death. Shortly afterwards, like his father, he married a commoner, Nefertiti, a woman with a reputation for shrewdness, who soon became his chief Queen. About six years into his reign (approximately 18 years old), for unknown reasons, Amenhotep IV changed his name to Akhenaten ("servant of Aten") and began to make plans for a grand new capitol city to be built on the east side of the Nile, 200 miles north of the capital, Thebes, on the west bank, in an area called Tell el-Amarna. Though his new city was called Akhetaten, this period of history is known as the Amarna era.

The religion of Egypt had always been polytheistic with numerous gods that had their respective spheres of responsibility for the activities of daily life, whether one was a common worker or the Pharoah. Reigning over all these deities, large and small, was Amun (or Amen), King of the Gods, and a powerful, extensive priestly class monitored adherence to the religious beliefs which covered every aspect of daily living from birth to death and from there the journey into the Afterlife. Egyptians of every social class from the king to the peasant believed in and relied upon magic in their daily lives. For such a great and extensive country, Egypt remained relatively stable[6] from the first Pharoah,[7] Narmer (3150 BC), to Amenhotep IV in 1350 BC, a period of 1800 years! However, this stability was unexpectedly shaken, not by a foreign enemy, epidemic, or other source, but by *an idea* that emanated from the throne; initiated by the Pharoah himself.

Perhaps the change of his name from Amenhotep IV to Akhenaten was influenced by his schooling in Heliopolis like other children of the upper classes, where the sun god, Ra, was venerated and depicted as a falcon-headed man with the disc of the sun on his head? It is obvious that he was taken with the solar aspects of the god because he transformed the god Ra by deleting the falcon-headed man, leaving only the disc of the sun, Aten, as the depersonalized god. Aten was seen as the creator of all that exists, especially the Nile River, and was the only God, "the living Aten beside whom there is no other; he was the sole god" (Redford, 1984, p. 171), and in reverence to this new god changed his name to Akhenaten ("servant of Aten"). Aten was represented by the disc of the sun with sunrays like long hands expanding downward and Akhenaten claimed that he was the only liaison between the one god, Aten, and his worshippers; like Moses was the interlocutor between God and the Israelites. He called the city he planned to build "Akhetaten" ("Horizon of Aten") and this project ultimately drained monies and workers away from the traditional capital of Thebes, likely embittering the established clergy and upper classes. As a further blow to the religious establishment, Akhenaten declared all other religions defunct and that

> Aten was not merely the supreme god, but the *only worshipable god*. He ordered the defacing of Amun's temples throughout Egypt and, in a number of instances, inscriptions of the plural 'gods' were also removed.
>
> (Ridley, 2019, p. 188) (italics added)

Akhenaten ascended to the throne when he was 12 years old, relocated the seat of power to Akhetaten (Amarna) six years later, and ruled for 17 years. His restrictions against praying to other gods grew increasingly harsh and reining in the power of the Amun priesthood brought on significant strife with great resentment of these constraints. He grew more enthralled in the promotion of his new religion, Atenism, while ignoring the quotidian requirements of the Pharoah, especially protecting the country from attacks by foreign adversaries on the periphery of Egyptian territory. Ultimately, with his death and the end of his rule, the pent-up bitterness of much of the population overflowed in a rampage to destroy what he had created: the city of Akhetaten was demolished, its buildings turned to rubble and carried off to Thebes for new building projects there; its temples ruined, and Akhenaten's name erased. The Priests of the old order returned, and the traditional gods were freely worshipped again. His son, Tutankhamen, became Pharoah at nine years old, reigned ten tumultuous years, and began to restore the old polytheistic order.

In *Moses and Monotheism*, Freud claimed that remnants of Atenism remained and that the "Moses" who was supposedly an Egyptian prince, and perhaps an adherent of Akhenaten's religion, adopted many aspects of that faith and blended these to create the beginnings of a new belief that would ultimately evolve into Judaism after a merger with the desert religion of Yahweh. However, Freud's assertion that Moses was an Egyptian and that Judaism developed out of Atenism has been met with considerable doubt and outright aggression, especially by Jews and Christians (see Rolnik, Chapter I). Redford (1996), for example, states that

> There is little or no evidence to support the notion that Akhenaten was a progenitor of the full-blown monotheism that we find in the Bible. The monotheism of the Hebrew Bible and the New Testament had its own separate development – *one that began more than half a millennium after the pharaoh's death.*
>
> (p. 179) (italics added)

I think that Freud might have responded to Redford's comment by reference to his writings about how traumatic events of a civilization may be repressed and remain latent until some subsequent event(s) triggers their emergence out of repression; a dynamic he had applied to the murder of Moses by the Israelites and the group's collective repression of that event. In this regard, Freud might have replied to Redford that the traumatic upheaval of Atenism was collectively repressed by Egyptian society and remained undiscovered for centuries, reawakened from its latent state after centuries of repose.

Freud was thrilled to hear of the excavations at Amarna and was disappointed that he was too old to undertake the physically taxing journey to that area of Egypt. He was, however, familiar with the writings of predecessors whose work influenced him, such as Friedrich Schiller's (1789) speculation "that Moses as the foster child of an Egyptian princess was initiated into a purely monotheistic Egyptian mystery religion which he subsequently taught to the Hebrews" (Yerushalmi, p. 5). In addition, Freud relied extensively on the work of the Biblical scholar Ernst Sellin (1922) who promulgated the theory that Moses never reached the Promised Land because he had been murdered by the resentful Israelites who could not tolerate the prophet's demand of adherence to his principles. These demands that there should be no belief in magic, that there was only one true god, that there should be no other gods before him, etc., were derivatives of Akhenaten's requirements on the Egyptian people which, according to Freud, seeded Moses' expectations of his followers.[8] In the end, both Akhenaten and Moses aspired to reach a Holy Land: Akhenaten's dream of a grand new city to honor his god, Aten, was realized for a precious few years: its wide boulevards, innovative architecture, numerous ateliers dedicated to the arts and temples of inventive design to the one God, Aten, graced this city of 30,000 (Seyfried, 2012) inhabitants until its destruction. In the Biblical version, Moses only got to look out over the Holy Land, but was kept from entering it and, in Freud's version, was murdered by his followers because, like Akhenaten, he demanded too much of them. Freud, on the other hand, identified with Moses and Akhenaten and had worried that his Amarna, psychoanalysis, would not flourish; that the Nazis, like the revanchist Priests of Egypt, would destroy his creation, psychoanalysis. *Moses and Monotheism* tells us the story of these three men, all heretics in their own right, and leaves us wondering, "What if all this is true?"

Notes

1 It was apparent by this time that Einstein's (1905) Special Theory of Relativity could open the possibility of a nuclear reaction that could be weaponized. Though avowedly a pacifist, but hearing of the Nazis' splitting of the atom in1938, Einstein was greatly alarmed and wrote a letter to President Roosevelt urging the development of a nuclear weapon. After the Second World War Einstein famously said, "I know not with what weapons World War III will be fought, but World War IV will be fought with sticks and stones."
2 The first temple in Jerusalem was built by King Solomon in 957 BC and was destroyed in 587 BC by the Babylonian King Nebuchadnezzer II. It was subsequently rebuilt in 515 BC and remained intact until it's destruction in 70 AD.
3 Germany's foreign policy during the Third Reich of Eastern expansion for more space required for life.
4 *Analysis Terminable and Interminable* (1937) and *An Outline of Psycho-Analysis* (1938).
5 *The Letters of Sigmund Freud and Arnold Zweig*, translated by W. D. Robson-Scott. London: Hogarth Press, 1970, p. 91.
6 The Hyksos conquered Northern Egypt and held it for about 100 years.
7 Narmer was anointed Pharoah (as opposed to King) because he joined Upper and Lower Egypt in 3150 BC.
8 Yerushalmi (1991), referring to the episode of the golden calf, quotes the Bible as saying that the Israelites said to Moses, "arise, make us a God (Exodus 32:1). Because he did not obey them, they stood over him and killed him." [This appears to come from a Midrash which is noted on p. 85 in Yerushalmi].

References

Andersen, E. (1998). The Rain Comes Down in Amsterdam. In *Memory of the Future.* Howie Epstein Studio, Beverly Hills, CA.

Assmann, J. (2014). *To Moses from Akhenaten: Ancient Egypt and Religious Change.* American University in Cairo Press. Cairo, Egypt.

Beier, M. (2020). Countering anti-semitism and religious violence: Freud and monotheism: Moses and the violent origins of religion. *Psa Rev* 107: 1–34.

Cohen, D. (2012). *The Escape of Sigmund Freud.* NY: The Overlook Press.

Einstein, A. (1933 [1932]). Letter to Sigmund Freud in *Why War*? SE:XXII, pp. 197–202.

Freud, S. (1915). Thoughts for the Times on War and Death. SE:XIV, pp. 273–301.
Freud, S. (1925). An Autobiographical Study. SE: 20, pp. 3–71.
Freud, S. (1927/1970). Letter to Arnold Zweig (2/7/27). In *The Letters of Arnold Zweig and Sigmund Freud*. Edited by Ernst L. Freud. NY: Harcourt, Brace & World.
Freud, S. (1930). *Civilization and Its Discontents*. SE: 21, pp. 59–147.
Freud, S. (1933 [1932]). Letter to Albert Einstein in *Why War?* SE: XXII, pp. 203–215.
Freud, S. (1937). *Constructions in Analysis*. SE: XXIII, pp. 255–270.
Freud, S. (1937). Letter to Ernst Jones, 2/3/1937. In *The Complete Correspondence of Sigmund Freud and Ernest Jones* 1908–1939. Edited by R. Andrew Paskauskas, 1993.
Freud, S. (1939). *Moses and Monotheism*. SE: XXIII. London: Hogarth Press.
Freud, S. (1940 [1938]) *An Outline of Psychoanalysis*. SE: XXIII, pp. 141–205.
Redford, D. (1984). *Akhenaten: The Heretic King*. Princeton University Press.
Redford, D. (1996). Aspects of Monotheism. *Biblical Archaeology Review*, 1996.
Ridley, T. (2019). *Akhenaten: A Historian's View*. The AUC History of Ancient Egypt. Cairo; New York: The American University in Cairo Press.
Sellin, E. (1922). *Mose und seine Bedeutung fur die israelitisch-judische Religionsgeschichte*. Leipzig and Erlangen: A. Deicherstsche Verlagsbuchhandlung.
Seyfried, F. (Ed.) (2012). *In the Light of Amarna: 100 Years of the Nefertiti Discovery*. Berlin: Agyptisches Museum und Papyrussammlung.
Yerushalmi, Y. H. (1991). Freud's *Moses: Judaism Terminable and Interminable*. New Haven: Yale University Press.

Index

For Product Safety Concerns and Information please contact our EU representative GPSR@taylorandfrancis.com
Taylor & Francis Verlag GmbH, Kaufingerstraße 24, 80331 München, Germany

www.ingramcontent.com/pod-product-compliance
Ingram Content Group UK Ltd.
Pitfield, Milton Keynes, MK11 3LW, UK
UKHW020140200926
475702UK00005B/837
9781032223124